THE COMPLETE GUIDE TO

YOGA

INVERSIONS

Learn How to Invert, Float, and Fly with Inversions and Arm Balances

JENNIFER DeCURTINS

FAIR WINDS

First published in the USA in 2015 by
Fair Winds Press, an imprint of
Quarto Publishing Group USA Inc.
100 Cummings Center
Suite 406-L
Beverly, MA 01915-6101
www.QuartoKnows.com
Visit our blogs at www.QuartoKnows.com

19 18 17 16 15   1 2 3 4 5

ISBN: 978-1-59233-694-4

Digital edition published in 2015
eISBN: 978-1-62788-759-5

Library of Congress Cataloging-in-Publication Data available

Cover and book design by Sporto
Photography by Wanda Koch

Printed and bound in China

*The information in this book is for educational purposes only. It is not
intended to replace the advice of a physician or medical practitioner. Please
see your health care provider before beginning any new health program.*

For my students, who are my greatest teachers.

CONTENTS

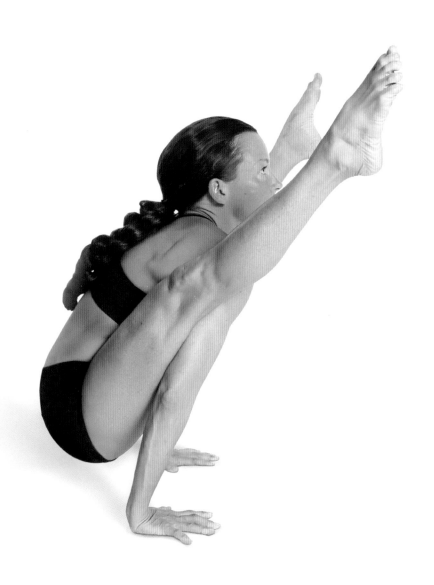

Introduction

Yoga can trace its roots back thousands of years and has experienced an evolution over time into many different lineages and styles. Yoga enjoys worldwide popularity for its numerous physical and emotional health benefits.

According to the 2013 "Yoga in America" study released by well-known yoga publication *Yoga Journal*, 20.4 million Americans practice yoga, and it's proven to be a growing trend. In 2008, the same study yielded 15.8 million participants. Over the course of five years, participation in yoga grew nearly 30 percent in the United States.

One of the appealing aspects of yoga is that it's accessible to everyone regardless of age or ability. Whether you're looking for a slow, restorative, meditative practice or a physical, challenging, fast-paced practice, there is a style of yoga to meet your needs.

In a typical yoga class, you perform a mixture of standing postures, balancing postures, backbends, inversions, twists, seated postures, and more. This combination of postures serves to strengthen and stretch your body while improving your mental state and enhancing focus and clarity.

This book explores how to take these common poses to uncommon places through inversions, arm balances, and advanced variations.

Benefits of Practicing Inversions, Arm Balances, and Advanced Asanas

Inversions, arm balances, and advanced asanas feature a variety of therapeutic benefits but are sometimes considered by students to be intimidating and out of reach. The thought of being upside down and balancing on the top of your head in headstand, kicking up to handstand, or supporting the weight of your body with only your arms in crow can be an overwhelming proposition at first.

But these postures are within reach. They simply require a willingness to try. It might not happen the first time, tenth time, or hundredth time you attempt the pose, but one day it will happen. Embrace being a little uncomfortable on your mat. Have a sense of humor and playfulness, and don't worry about what you look like attempting the pose or if you fall or wobble trying.

One of the most amazing things about yoga is the transformation that occurs on the mat when you show up and dedicate yourself to the practice. The body and mind begin to open in a way that they never have before. You open to possibility, growth, and change. After maintaining a regular practice for a period of time, most students find themselves performing postures they once were certain they would never do.

Through practice and trust, inversions, arm balances, and advanced asanas are within reach. Mastering them often brings with it a tremendous amount of confidence and marks a milestone in one's personal practice.

INVERSIONS

The term "inversion" simply means having the head lower than the heart. Inversions have physical, psychological, and emotional benefits.

Physically, they strengthen the arms, legs, and core muscles while also helping to improve posture by focusing on midline stability. Going upside down also helps return blood flow back to the heart, which improves circulation and blood flow to the brain. This also helps with tired, swollen legs and ankles when applied in a feet-up-the-wall type of scenario.

Psychologically, these postures can both energize and heat the body and also cool and relax the nervous system, depending on the type of inversion. Inversions can help with stress management and insomnia.

Emotionally, inversions help with overcoming fear and doubt and building self-confidence and body awareness.

ARM BALANCES

The term "arm balance" means any pose that requires you to balance on your arms/hands with no other body part touching the ground. These poses require a combination of strength and flexibility.

Physically, arm balances are especially beneficial for building core and upper body strength. They are weight-bearing poses that can help prevent osteoporosis. Arm balances also help to improve balance and coordination, which are essential functional movements for all aging adults.

Emotionally, like inversions, arm balances are major fear busters and can open you up to believe in your body's ability and strength.

ADVANCED ASANAS

The advanced asanas in this book can't be categorized as arm balances or inversions, but they offer deeper and more challenging variations of traditional poses. These asanas help you explore the playful nature of your practice.

This book features a collection of more than 125 inversions, arm balances, and advanced asanas that are found in a variety of styles of yoga including Ashtanga, Bikram, power, hatha, and more.

The book is broken into five sections: foundational poses, standing poses, balancing poses, inverted poses, and seated poses. Each section features "gateway" poses that are common to a typical yoga class. The book will guide you through progressions of the gateway pose into more advanced inversions, arm balances, and other asanas.

The goal of this book is to inspire students to see the possibility that exists with their personal practice and to serve as a guide for teachers to assist with incorporating inversions, arm balances, and advanced asanas into their classes and sequencing.

1

Foundational Poses

Almost every yoga practice includes the basic postures found in this section: down dog, side plank, three point, forward fold, wide leg forward fold, garland, dolphin, and wheel. Although relatively simple in their basic form, these poses can take you to new places in your practice.

Imagine floating into a handstand from down dog, coming into full wheel from three point, or finding firefly pose from a wide leg forward fold. The possibilities are endless when you open your mind and your practice to the idea that the basics don't have to be boring.

In this section, you will learn how to advance your basic asana with inversions, arm balances, backbends, and many places between!

GATEWAY POSE:

DOWN DOG *(Adho Mukha Svanasana)*

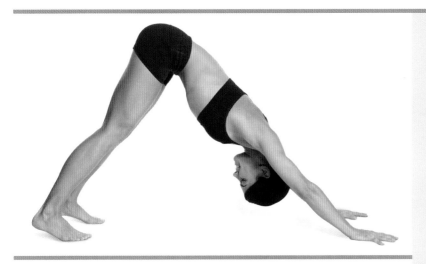

Down dog (or downward facing dog) is one of the most basic poses in yoga. It's actually a gentle inversion in itself as your hips are elevated higher than your head. This is a pose you'll come back to throughout the course of a class. It's a great check-in pose that allows you to scan your body from head to toes to take inventory of what feels tight, heavy, and in need of stretching and breath.

Down dog is a great pose for transitioning from the top to the back of the mat, and it's used in everything from sun salutations to power flow sequences. It serves as a gateway pose into poses as basic as half dog to as advanced as handstand.

HOW TO GET THERE:

- Start in high plank with your shoulders stacked directly over your wrists.
- Lift your hips up and back as you come into an upside-down V position.

WHERE TO ENGAGE:

- Press firmly into your palms, grounding them down into the mat. Especially focus on the spot between your thumb and first finger.
- Keep your arms long and straight and your shoulders away from your ears.
- Draw your navel in and up, and pull your chest back toward your thighs.
- Squeeze through your quads to sink your heels down into the mat, pressing the back of your thighs toward the back of the room.

ANATOMY NOTES/ TIPS & TRICKS:

- It's common to want to shorten down dog to get your heels to touch the floor. Check yourself by shifting back out to high plank. Your shoulders should still stack over your wrists without you having to walk your hands back.
- Focus on rotating your upper arms inward to pull your shoulders away from your ears.
- Focus on spiraling your outer thighs away from one another to prevent your feet from caving in.
- Gaze back between your knees or up toward your navel.

DOWN DOG ADVANCED ASANA:
HALF DOG *(Uttana Shishosana)*

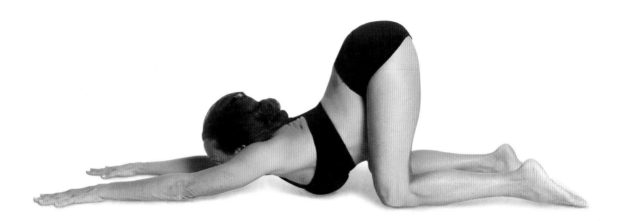

HOW TO GET THERE:

- Begin in down dog, and drop down to your knees.

- Keep your hips stacked directly over your knees, and extend your arms out toward the front of the mat.

- Rest your forehead, chin, or chest on the floor.

WHERE TO ENGAGE:

- Press through your palms as you pull your chest down toward the floor and your shoulder blades down your back.

- Draw your navel in toward your spine, engaging through your belly.

- Lift upward through your hips.

ANATOMY NOTES/ TIPS & TRICKS:

- Resist the urge to sit back toward child's pose, and keep your hips directly over your knees.

- Don't worry about whether your forehead, chin, or chest touch the floor. All are correct variations.

DOWN DOG INVERSION:
JUMP TO HANDSTAND

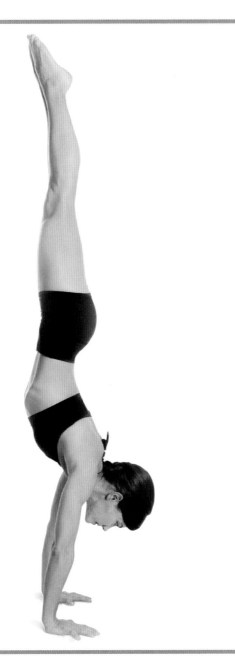

HOW TO GET THERE:

- Begin in down dog.

- Take a deep bend in the knees, bringing your shins parallel to the mat.

- Look between your hands, and jump toward the top of the mat, stacking your hips over your shoulders to press into handstand.

WHERE TO ENGAGE:

- Powerfully explode (or push) through the legs as you jump forward and up to bring your hips over your shoulders.

- Squeeze your inner thighs in together as you come into handstand while keeping your core tight and engaged.

- Press into your fingertips and palms to find balance.

ANATOMY NOTES/ TIPS & TRICKS:

- Practice this by working repetitions of jumping to the top of the mat and stacking your hips over your shoulders. Don't even worry about the actual handstand until you can get some airtime here.

- Look to the top of the mat before you jump forward. Always look toward your target!

- Look between your hands to your fingertips once you're in handstand.

DOWN DOG ARM BALANCE:
JUMP TO CROW *(Bakasana)*

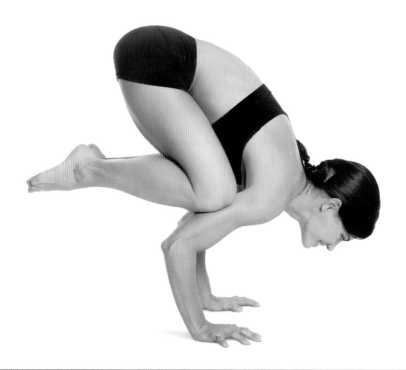

HOW TO GET THERE:

- Begin in down dog.
- Take a deep bend in your knees, bringing your shins parallel to the mat.
- Look between your hands, and jump toward the top of the mat, drawing your knees in toward your chest.
- Lightly land your knees on top of your triceps to come into crow pose.

WHERE TO ENGAGE:

- Explode through your legs as you jump forward and up to bring your hips over your shoulders.
- Draw your knees up your triceps, lift your heels up toward your butt, and be strong in your core in crow pose.
- Press into your fingertips and palms to find balance.

ANATOMY NOTES/ TIPS & TRICKS:

- Really focus on feeling light here as you jump your knees onto your triceps. Maintain as much upward lift as you can as you jump and balance in crow.
- Gaze forward through your hands as you jump and in front of your fingertips in crow.

DOWN DOG ADVANCED ASANA:
MAD DOG

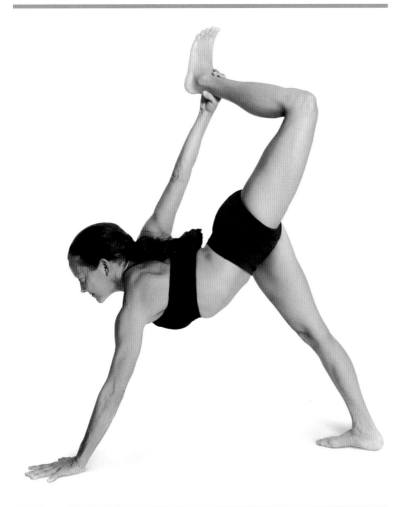

HOW TO GET THERE:

- Begin in down dog.

- Bend your left knee, and reach your right hand back for the inside of your left ankle.

- Keep your hips and shoulders square to the mat as you balance in this bind.

WHERE TO ENGAGE:

- Press firmly through the grounded palm to stabilize your shoulder.

- Scoop your chest through your shoulders, and draw your belly in and up.

- Kick your hand and foot together, and lift your bent knee upward, engaging through your quad.

ANATOMY NOTES/ TIPS & TRICKS:

- This one requires a lot of balance and breath! Take it easy and slow.

- Gaze out in front of your hands.

GATEWAY POSE:
THREE POINT

Three point is a simple variation of down dog. While often used for lunging a leg to the top of the mat, three point can also take you into everything from backbends to arm balances. The lifted leg gives you momentum and leverage to move into poses such as full wheel, mountain climber, chin stand, revolved side plank, and more.

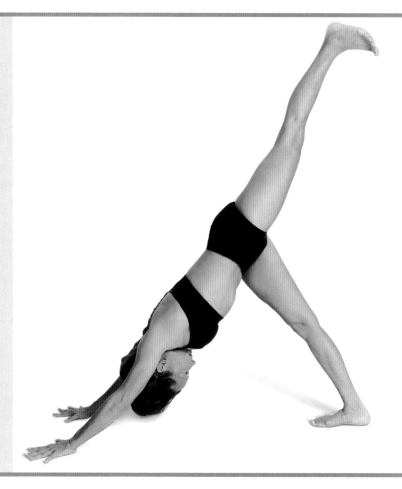

HOW TO GET THERE:

- Begin in down dog.
- Bring your big toes together to touch and lift one leg straight up in the air behind you.

WHERE TO ENGAGE:

- Spread your fingertips wide, and press firmly into your palms with equal pressure in both palms, and keep your shoulders square to the mat. Keep your arms long and straight.
- Sink your grounded heel down toward the mat.
- Squeeze through the lifted leg, keeping it straight and pointing your toes.

ANATOMY NOTES/ TIPS & TRICKS:

- It's common in three point to want to rotate your lifted hip open to lift your leg higher. Keep your hip as square to the floor as possible, even if it means you can't lift your leg as high.
- Gaze back toward the navel or lifted leg.

THREE POINT ADVANCED ASANA:
BOUND REVOLVED SIDE PLANK

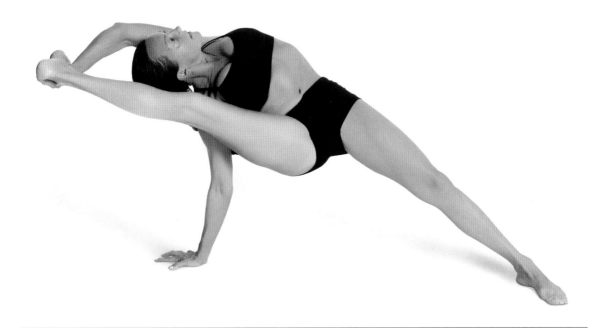

HOW TO GET THERE:

- Begin in three point.

- Draw your right knee into your chest and as you do, spin the blade of your left foot flat, and shift your weight onto your right hand, similar to how you would for a side plank.

- Grab the outside of your right foot with your left hand, and reach through your right heel to straighten your leg.

WHERE TO ENGAGE:

- Ground down through your left foot to anchor and support your body.

- Press firmly into your right palm to lift up through your side body.

- Reach through your heel, and try to rotate your upper body open toward the ceiling with your gaze under your left arm.

ANATOMY NOTES/ TIPS & TRICKS:

- Don't worry so much about straightening the extended leg. Focus more on reaching through your heel to lengthen your hamstring.

- Keep your focus on pressing down through your palm to twist open to the ceiling. Point your chest and gaze to the ceiling.

- If you need more support starting out, place your left foot against a wall to provide more grounding and stability.

- Release your right foot from your left hand, return your left hand to the mat, and lift your right leg back up to three point to exit the advanced asana.

THREE POINT ADVANCED ASANA:
FLIP DOG

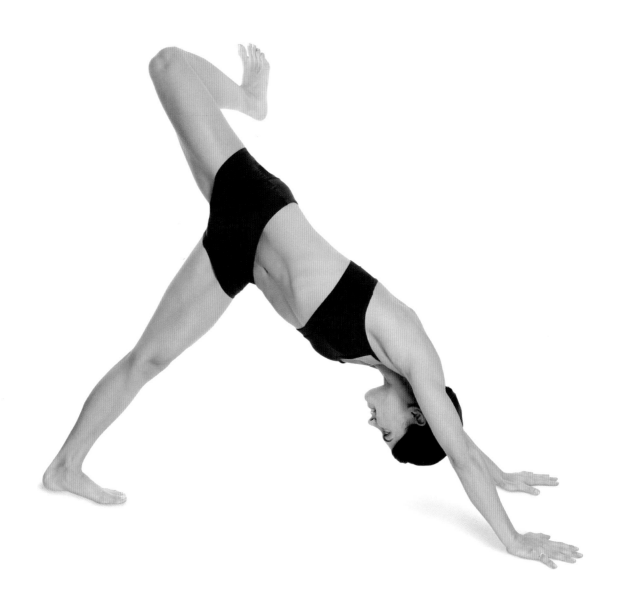

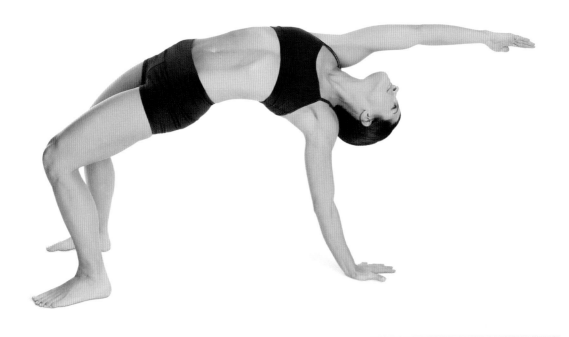

HOW TO GET THERE:

- Begin in three point.

- Take a bend in your right knee. Point your knee toward the ceiling, stack your hips, and let your heel hang down toward your gluteus.

- Shift your weight onto your left hand, lift your right hand off the mat, and let the momentum of your right heel hanging bring you into a backbend position with both heels flat on the floor.

WHERE TO ENGAGE:

- Press into your heels to lift your hips.

- Let your head fall back and your chest and neck stretch open.

- Press firmly into your grounded left palm to support the weight of your body.

ANATOMY NOTES/ TIPS & TRICKS:

- Keep your hips lifted as much as possible during the transition from three point to flip dog. Try to avoid dipping your hips and glutes down toward the mat before you come into the backbend. Think about maintaining an arc position throughout.

- This is a nice variation of three point that feels great, looks fun, and is beginner friendly.

THREE POINT ARM BALANCE:
MOUNTAIN CLIMBER

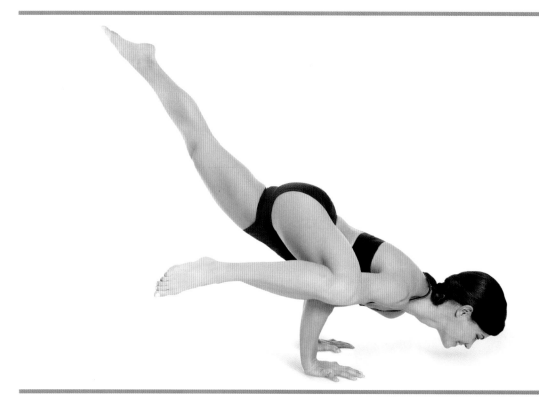

HOW TO GET THERE:

- Begin in three point.

- Bring your right knee to the outside of your right tricep. As you do so, shift your weight forward so that your shoulders begin to stack over your wrists.

- Bend your elbows to 90 degrees, squeeze them into your side body as if you were performing a chaturanga, and place your right knee on your right tricep.

- Shift your weight forward onto your fingertips, and lift up through your left leg.

WHERE TO ENGAGE:

- Press firmly into your palms, and really grip into your fingertips, bringing more weight forward than feels comfortable.

- Reach forward with your chest as you squeeze in through your elbows.

- Squeeze through the straightened lifted leg.

ANATOMY NOTES/ TIPS & TRICKS:

- Shorten your down dog when you go into three point to make it easier to get your right knee to the outside of your right tricep.

- When you first start with this arm balance, you may keep your chin down on the floor. That is okay, but avoid turning to the side of your head and resting on your cheek for the safety of your neck. As you progress, try to lift your chin off the floor.

- Momentum is your friend here. Once you start to move forward, use your forward momentum to launch you into your arm balance.

- To exit the arm balance, lunge your left leg back, and lift your right leg to three point.

THREE POINT ARM BALANCE:
REVOLVED MOUNTAIN CLIMBER

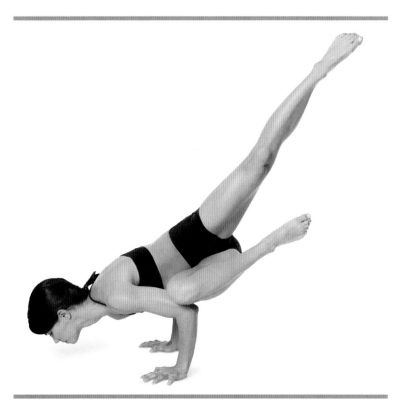

ANATOMY NOTES/ TIPS & TRICKS:

- When you first start out, you may keep your chin down on the floor. That's okay, but avoid turning to the side of your head and resting on your cheek for the safety of your neck. As you progress, try to lift your chin off the floor.

- When you first start out, you may ground your right hip on your right elbow, but as you become more comfortable with the arm balance, you can play with lifting your hips higher than your elbow to give you more leverage to move around.

- Momentum is your friend here. Once you start to move forward and twist, use your forward momentum to launch you into your arm balance.

- To exit the arm balance, lunge your left leg back, untwist, and lift your right leg to three point.

HOW TO GET THERE:

- Begin in three point.

- Bring your right knee across your chest toward your left tricep. As you do so, shift your weight forward so that your shoulders begin to stack over your wrists.

- Bend your elbows to 90 degrees, squeeze them into your side as if you were performing a chaturanga, and place your right knee on your left tricep.

- Shift your weight forward onto your fingertips, and lift up through your left leg.

WHERE TO ENGAGE:

- Press firmly into your palms, and really grip into your fingertips, bringing more weight forward than feels comfortable.

- Reach forward with your chest as you squeeze in through your elbows.

- A deep spinal twist with engaged abs is required to get your knee to your opposite tricep and to launch into your arm balance.

- Squeeze through the straightened lifted leg.

THREE POINT ARM BALANCE:
DOUBLE LEG MOUNTAIN CLIMBER OR CHIN STAND

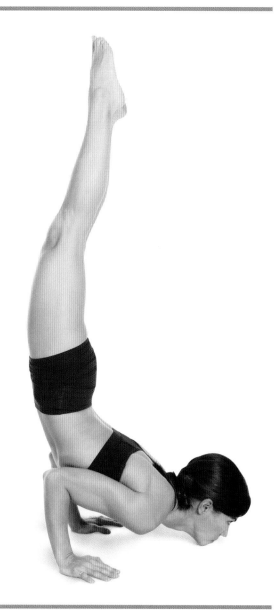

HOW TO GET THERE:

- Begin in three point, and move into mountain climber with your right knee on your right tricep.

- Keep your elbows glued to your side body at a 90 degree bend as you press into your fingertips and lift your right leg off of your right tricep and up to meet your left.

- Squeeze your legs together overhead in a straight line, and point your toes.

WHERE TO ENGAGE:

- Press firmly into your palms, and really grip into your fingertips, bringing more weight forward than feels comfortable.

- Reach forward with your chest as you squeeze in through your elbows, and allow your chin to rest lightly on the floor with your gaze forward.

- Abdominal engagement is key for lifting from mountain climber to straight legs. Squeeze everything in!

ANATOMY NOTES/TIPS & TRICKS:

- Your chin can rest on the floor in this arm balance, but avoid turning to the side of your face to keep your neck safe.

- Maintain a straight line from heel to hip to elbow, and avoid letting your lower back arch by keeping your abs engaged.

- The hardest part of this arm balance is lifting from mountain climber to straight legs. Once you have your legs straight overhead, this is relatively simple to hold.

- Lunge your left leg back, and lift your right leg to three point to exit the arm balance.

THREE POINT ARM BALANCE:
SCORPION DOUBLE-LEG MOUNTAIN CLIMBER OR SCORPION CHIN STAND

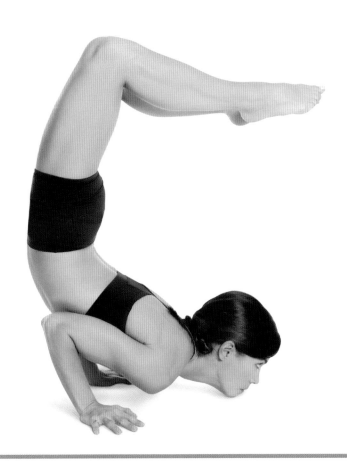

- Keep reaching through your heels toward your head to deepen your backbend.

ANATOMY NOTES/ TIPS & TRICKS:

- Your chin can rest on the floor in this arm balance, but avoid turning to the side of your face to keep your neck safe.

- Maintain a straight line from hips to elbows, and make sure your backbend is coming from reaching through your chest and not putting stress on your lower back.

- Straighten your legs, lunge your left leg back, and lift your right leg to three point to exit the arm balance.

HOW TO GET THERE:

- Begin in double leg mountain climber/chin stand.

- Keep your elbows glued to your side body as you press into your fingertips.

- Bend your knees, and bring your heels overhead.

WHERE TO ENGAGE:

- Press firmly into your palms, and really grip into your fingertips, bringing more weight forward than feels comfortable.

- Reach forward with your chest as you squeeze in through your elbows, and allow your chin to rest lightly on the floor with your gaze forward.

GATEWAY POSE:

SIDE PLANK *(Vasisthasana)*

Side plank is commonly used in yoga classes as a pose to develop core strength, especially in the side body and obliques. Side plank is also a great pose to use to transition from one pose to another— for example, side angle to side plank to high plank to down dog.

In its simplest form, side plank has you maintain a straight body position while balancing on one hand and one foot. Once you feel comfortable and stable holding side plank, have a little fun mixing it up with some more challenging options.

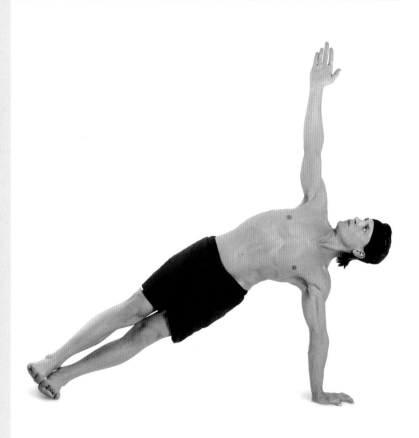

HOW TO GET THERE:

- Start in high plank with your shoulders stacked directly over your wrists.

- Roll to one side (either right or left), stack your shoulder over your wrist, and extend your top hand straight up toward the ceiling.

- Stack your hips and feet on top of one another.

WHERE TO ENGAGE:

- Press firmly into the grounded palm to stabilize through your shoulder.

- Lift up through your hips like you're trying to create a C-shape in your side body.

- Squeeze through your core and legs to help your body feel strong and supported in the pose.

ANATOMY NOTES/ TIPS & TRICKS:

- Split your feet on the floor instead of stacking for a little more support and stability.

- Gaze straight ahead or up toward your lifted hand.

- The lifted arm can be extended over your head, bringing your bicep over your ear for more extension through your side body.

SIDE PLANK ADVANCED ASANA:
TREE SIDE PLANK

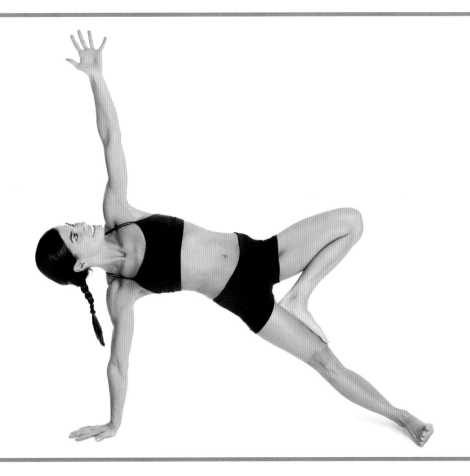

HOW TO GET THERE:

- Begin in side plank.

- Bend your top knee, and place the sole of your foot on the inside of the shin or thigh of your grounded leg with your knee pointing to the ceiling to find a tree pose in side plank.

WHERE TO ENGAGE:

- Press firmly into the grounded palm to stabilize through your shoulder.

- Lift up through your hips toward the ceiling.

- Firmly press your foot into your thigh to provide leverage and stability in the pose.

ANATOMY NOTES/ TIPS & TRICKS:

- Gaze straight ahead or up toward the ceiling.

- Don't let your top knee cave inward in tree pose. Actively press it back.

- Avoid placing your foot directly on your knee joint. Make sure it's on your shin or thigh.

- Your top arm can reach straight up or extend over your head, bringing your bicep over your ear for extra side body lengthening.

SIDE PLANK ADVANCED ASANA:
STAR SIDE PLANK

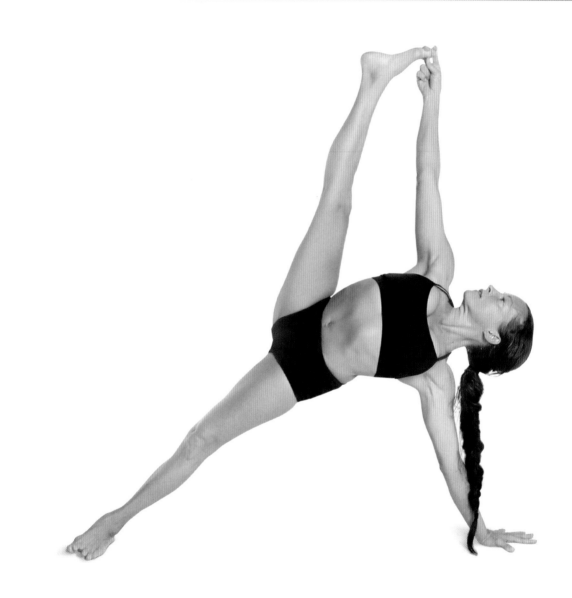

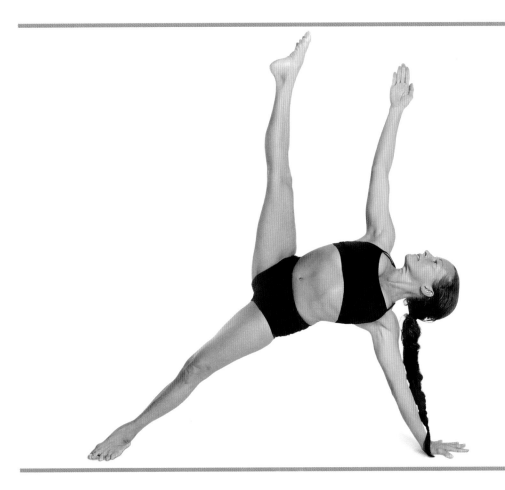

HOW TO GET THERE:

- Begin in side plank.

- Bend your top knee, and bring the knee in toward your chest. Hook your index and middle fingers around your big toe, and straighten your leg toward the ceiling.

- Pull your right toes back, and reach through your heel. Feel the right side of your body lift upward.

WHERE TO ENGAGE:

- Press firmly into the grounded palm to stabilize through your shoulder.

- Squeeze through the quadriceps of the extended leg to lengthen your hamstring and straighten your leg.

ANATOMY NOTES/ TIPS & TRICKS:

- Gaze up toward the lifted leg.

- Make sure you feel your fingertips pressing down into the mat to prevent placing all your weight in your palm and compressing your wrist.

- For an extra core challenge, release your toes, and let the extended leg hover in the star position.

SIDE PLANK ADVANCED ASANA:
BOW/BOUND SIDE PLANK

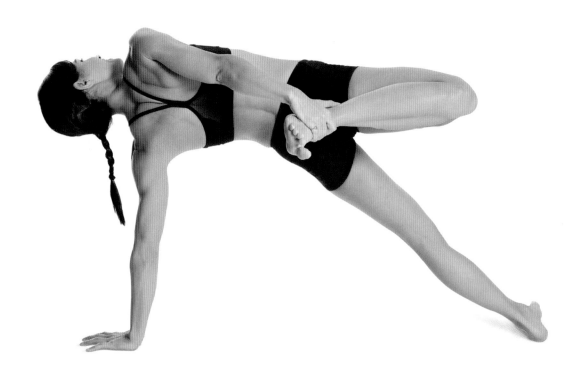

HOW TO GET THERE:

- Begin in side plank.

- Draw your top knee in toward your chest, and wrap your lifted hand around your ankle or top of your foot.

- Kick your hand and foot together to press your heel back behind you while opening your chest and lifting through your hips. It's a half bow pose in side plank.

WHERE TO ENGAGE:

- Press firmly into your grounded hand to stabilize through your shoulder and to lift up through your hips.

- Firmly kick your hand and foot together to help open into the bow pose.

ANATOMY NOTES/ TIPS & TRICKS:

- Gaze straight ahead or lifted toward the ceiling.

- Your chest can face forward or rotate open toward the ceiling.

SIDE PLANK ADVANCED ASANA:
KASYAPASANA

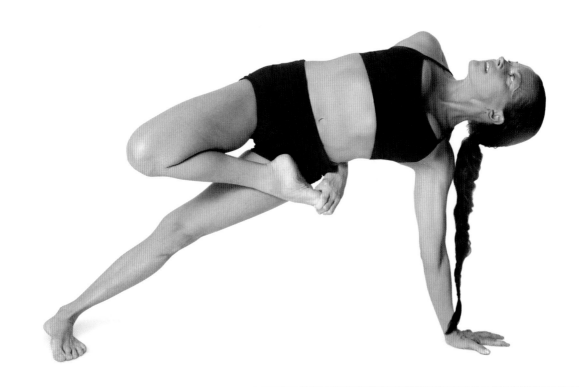

HOW TO GET THERE:

- Begin in a seated position, and draw your right foot into your left leg with the blade of your foot tucked into the crease of your left thigh to find lotus.

- Reach your right hand behind your back, and take hold of the top of your right foot.

- Place your left palm flat on the floor with your fingers facing away. Begin to roll to the left to come into side plank with the lotus bind.

WHERE TO ENGAGE:

- Press into your grounded hand for stabilization.

- As you lift your side body, ground down through the instep of your left foot.

ANATOMY NOTES/ TIPS & TRICKS:

- Gaze straight ahead or toward the ceiling.

- Your ultimate goal is to rotate your chest toward the ceiling while lifting your hips as high as possible.

GATEWAY POSE:
DOLPHIN

Dolphin is essentially down dog on your forearms. This variation of down dog is used to deepen the opening of your upper thoracic spine, while improving shoulder stability and stretching your latissimus dorsi and triceps.

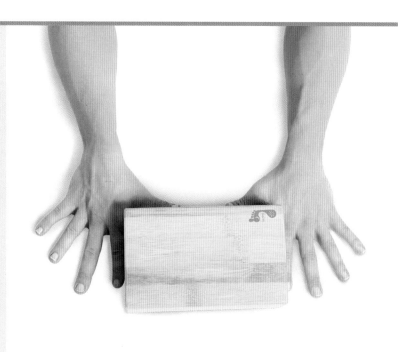

HOW TO GET THERE:

- Begin in down dog.
- One arm at a time, lower down to your forearms.

WHERE TO ENGAGE:

- Spread your fingers wide, and press down through your forearms.
- Press your chest back toward your thighs.

- Engage your quadriceps to lengthen though your hamstrings while also pressing your heels down toward the mat.

ANATOMY NOTES/ TIPS & TRICKS:

- Wrists and elbows should be in line with your shoulders. There is a tendency for your hands to slide in toward one another and your elbows to slide away from one another.

- Use a block to help you maintain proper alignment. Make an L-shape with your pointer finger and thumb, and place the block flat and horizontal in the space between your hands.

- Gaze back between your knees or between your forearms. Keep your neck relaxed, and draw your shoulders down away from your ears.

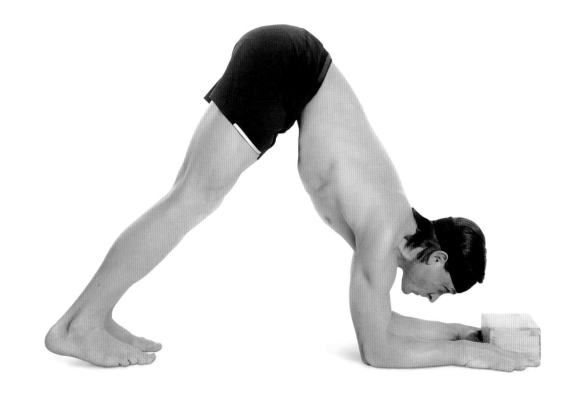

DOLPHIN ARM BALANCE/INVERSION:
FOREARM BALANCE *(Pincha Mayurasana)*

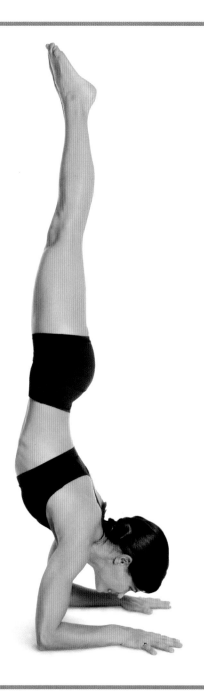

HOW TO GET THERE:

- Begin in dolphin, and walk your feet in closer to your elbows.

- Shift your gaze forward between your hands.

- Lift your right leg straight up, and come high onto your left toes until your right hip is stacked over your shoulders.

- Lift your left leg up to meet your right, forming a straight line from your toes to your elbows.

WHERE TO ENGAGE:

- Spread your fingers wide, and press down through your forearms.

- Engage your abdominals, gluteus, and inner thighs to stabilize once you are completely inverted.

ANATOMY NOTES/
TIPS & TRICKS:

- Your wrists and elbows should be in line with your shoulders. There is a tendency for your hands to slide in toward one another and your elbows to slide away from one another.

- You can use a block to help you maintain proper alignment. Make L-shapes with your pointer fingers and thumbs, and place the block flat and horizontal in the space between your hands.

- Initially, you can gaze down to the floor or at your fingertips until you feel comfortable in the pose. Eventually, gaze back behind you with your head straight down toward the floor.

- Do not rely on momentum to get into this posture. Practice controlling the lift of your legs rather than trying to jump or kick into the inversion.

DOLPHIN ARM BALANCE/INVERSION:
SCORPION *(Vrischikasana I)*

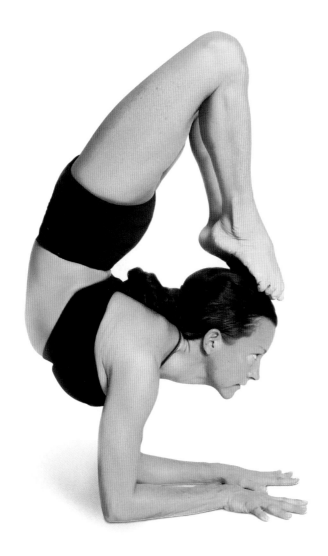

HOW TO GET THERE:

- Begin in forearm balance.

- Take your gaze forward, looking straight out in front of you.

- Pull your chest through your shoulders as you bend both knees and reach the tips of your toes toward the back of your head.

WHERE TO ENGAGE:

- Spread your fingers wide, and press down through your forearms.

- Squeeze your hamstrings to get your toes closer to the back of your head.

ANATOMY NOTES/ TIPS & TRICKS:

- Your wrists and elbows should be in line with your shoulders. There is a tendency for your hands to slide in toward one another and your elbows to slide away from one another.

- Use a block to help you maintain proper alignment. Make L-shapes with your pointer fingers and thumbs, and place the block flat and horizontal in the space between your hands.

- When you lift your gaze forward, be mindful to keep your neck long.

GATEWAY POSE:
FORWARD FOLD *(Ragdoll)*

Forward folds are one of the most basic yoga poses, but the benefits of this simple posture are numerous. First and foremost, they are great for relieving tight hamstrings and helping with lower back pain. They are also gentle inversions and are very calming for the brain, helping to relieve stress, headaches, anxiety, insomnia, and more.

In this gateway pose, we will explore how different hand positions can change and bring variety to your forward fold as well as how to move into arm balances and inversions from a forward fold.

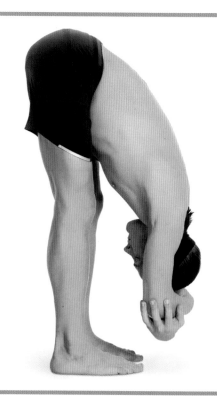

HOW TO GET THERE:

- Begin in a standing position with your feet hip distance apart.

- With your knees slightly bent, hinge at your waist, fold forward, and allow your head to hang down toward the floor.

- Keep your knees slightly bent, and take your opposite elbows in your hand, allowing your head to hang in the space between your arms with your neck completely relaxed.

WHERE TO ENGAGE:

- Draw your navel in and up toward your spine to protect your lower back and facilitate a deeper fold.

ANATOMY NOTES/ TIPS & TRICKS:

- While your hamstrings receive a gentle stretch in forward fold, the emphasis in this pose is more on opening your lower back.

- Many students tend to want to look at their toes, but take your gaze back between your legs to keep your neck long.

- Once you get into the pose, it feels good to sway your upper body side to side to further open and stretch your lower back.

FORWARD FOLD ADVANCED ASANA:
BIG TOES *(Padangusthasana)*

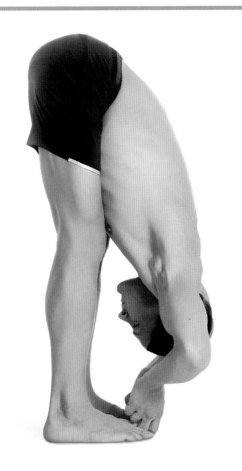

HOW TO GET THERE:

- Begin in a standing position with your feet hip distance apart.

- With your knees slightly bent, hinge at your waist, fold forward, and allow your head to hang down toward the floor.

- Wrap your index and middle fingers around your big toes. While still holding your toes, lift your chest as high as you can to lengthen your spine. Keep your knees slightly bent as you do this. Fold forward once again, and reach the crown of your head toward the floor.

WHERE TO ENGAGE:

- Draw your navel in and up toward your spine to protect your lower back and create the space to fold deeper.

- Flex your abdominal muscles to help release through your lower back.

- Squeeze through your quadriceps to stretch deeper into your hamstrings.

ANATOMY NOTES/
TIPS & TRICKS:

- Shift weight out of your heels and more onto the balls of your feet to stack your hips over your ankles.

- Visualize your hips lifting up as the crown of your head reaches down, and gaze back between your legs to keep your neck long and relaxed.

- Notice if the arches of your feet are collapsing. If so, roll weight to the outside blades of your feet to lift them up.

FORWARD FOLD ADVANCED ASANA:
GORILLA *(Padhahastasana)*

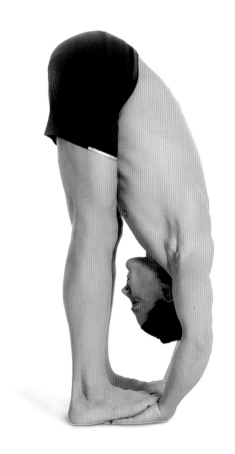

HOW TO GET THERE:

• Begin in a standing position with your feet hip distance apart.

• With your knees slightly bent, hinge at your waist, fold forward, and allow your head to hang down toward the floor.

• Lift your gaze, lengthen your spine, and slide your hands under your feet with your palms facing up. Fold forward once again.

• Bend your knees as much as you need to get your toes to your wrists.

WHERE TO ENGAGE:

• Draw your navel in and up toward your spine to protect your lower back and create the space to fold deeper.

• Flex your abdominal muscles to help release through your lower back.

• Squeeze through your quadriceps to stretch deeper into your hamstrings.

ANATOMY NOTES/
TIPS & TRICKS:

• Shift weight out of your heels and more onto the balls of your feet to stack your hips over your ankles.

• Visualize your hips lifting up as the crown of your head reaches down, and gaze back between your legs to keep your neck long and relaxed.

FORWARD FOLD ADVANCED ASANA:
BINDING SHOULDER OPENER

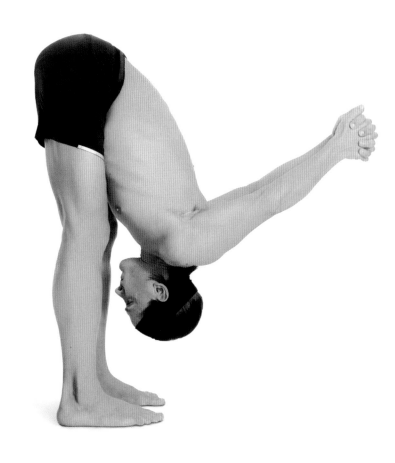

HOW TO GET THERE:

- Begin in a standing position with your feet hip distance apart.

- Interlace your hands together behind your back.

- With your knees slightly bent, hinge at your waist, fold forward, and allow your head to hang down toward the floor. Keeping the bind, reach your arms over your head.

WHERE TO ENGAGE:

- Draw your navel in and up toward your spine to protect your lower back and create the space to fold deeper.

- Keep your palms squeezed in as closely as possible as you reach your arms over your head.

- Squeeze through your quadriceps to stretch deeper into your hamstrings.

ANATOMY NOTES/
TIPS & TRICKS:

- Shift weight out of your heels and more onto the balls of your feet to stack your hips over your ankles.

- The tendency is to want to separate your palms as you fold forward to get your arms further over your head, but keep them together and touching if possible.

- If your shoulders are too tight to bind, use a towel or a strap.

FORWARD FOLD ADVANCED ASANA:
BIND BEHIND THE BACK *(Titibasana B)*

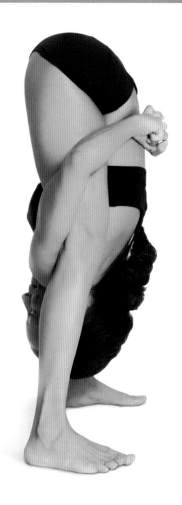

HOW TO GET THERE:

- Begin in one of the forward folds previously listed, and release any bind you may have.

- Keeping your knees bent as much as you need, and with one arm at a time, begin to work one shoulder behind your leg followed by the other, positioning each leg as far up onto your tricep as possible.

- Once both your shoulders are behind your legs, relax your head down.

- Reach one arm behind your back and as far up your back as possible, allowing your shoulder to internally rotate as you do so.

- Repeat for your other arm.

- Once both are behind your back, interlace your fingers, taking a bind.

- After your bind is secure, begin to straighten your legs as much as you can.

WHERE TO ENGAGE:

- Draw your navel in and up toward your spine to protect your lower back and create the space to fold deeper.

- Flex your abdominal muscles to help release through your lower back.

- Squeeze through your quadriceps to stretch deeper into your hamstrings.

ANATOMY NOTES/TIPS & TRICKS:

- Once your lower back is open enough to explore this variation, the next biggest challenge is the bind. The key to taking a bind is to relax as much as you can while doing so. The more you try to engage while searching for the bind, the more difficult it will be.

- Shift weight out of your heels and more onto the balls of your feet to stack your hips over your ankles.

- If your shoulders are too tight to bind, use a towel or strap.

FORWARD FOLD ARM BALANCE:
CROW *(Bakasana)*

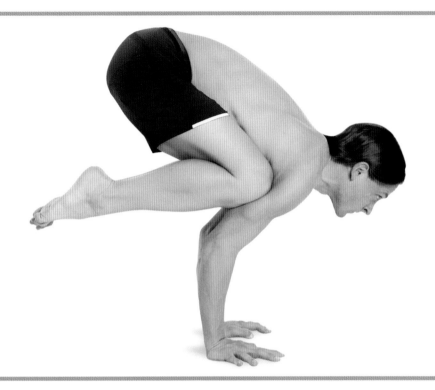

HOW TO GET THERE:

- Begin in one of the forward folds on pages 34–37, and release any bind you may have.

- Bring your palms to the floor, and begin to bend your knees and your elbows.

- Stack your knees on top of your triceps as close to your armpits as possible. Bring your toes together to touch.

- Shift your weight forward, and lift your toes off the floor.

WHERE TO ENGAGE:

- Bring a lot of weight forward and really press into your palms, grip into your fingertips, and lift up through your chest.

- Squeeze your elbows in like you would in a chaturanga, staying very active in your arms.

- Think heels to butt, and really lift up through your legs.

- Draw your abdominal wall in and up to help support the weight of your body in the arm balance.

ANATOMY NOTES/ TIPS & TRICKS:

- Shift more weight forward than you think is necessary, and feel the weight in your palms and fingertips.

- Envision your whole body engaging and lifting up. Nothing should be loose or disengaged here.

- If you are struggling with your arm balance, place your feet on a block and your palms on the floor. This helps get you into the proper position for crow, and you can begin to practice lifting one foot off the block and then two for the arm balance.

FORWARD FOLD INVERSION:
HANDSTAND PRESS

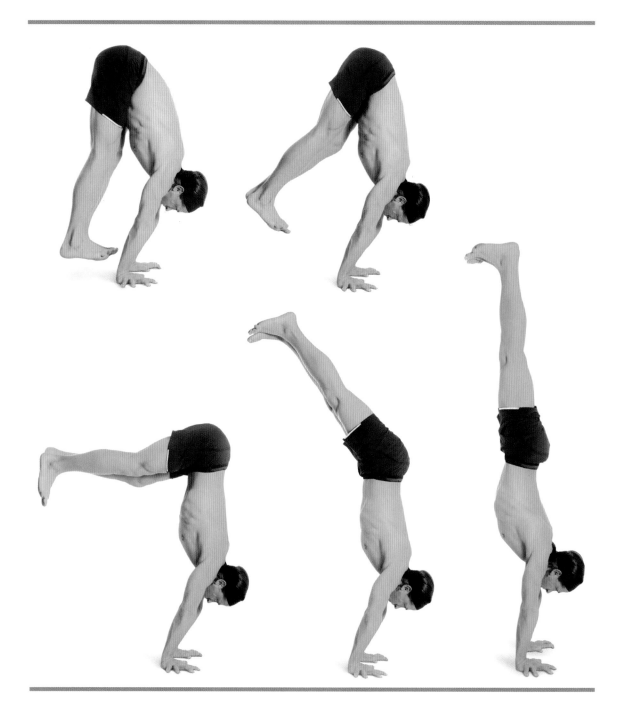

HOW TO GET THERE:

- Begin in one of the forward folds on pages 34–37, and release any bind you may have.

- Lift your gaze, lengthen your spine, and place your hands flat on the floor.

- Keep your gaze lifted, looking between your hands and coming high onto your toes, while keeping your elbows fully extended and your shoulders externally rotated for stability.

- Shift your weight onto your hands until your toes leave the floor and your hips come slightly in front of your shoulders.

- As you lift your legs upwards, your hips will continue to shift even more forward in front of your shoulders until your legs are parallel to the floor.

- Once your legs are above parallel, gradually shift your hips back over your shoulders until they align.

WHERE TO ENGAGE:

- Actively flex your abdominal muscles to prevent backward momentum and your gluteus maximus to prevent yourself from folding forward at your waist and coming down.

- Engage your triceps to keep your elbows in full extension.

- Squeeze your inner thighs to keep your legs together.

ANATOMY NOTES/ TIPS & TRICKS:

- The goal is to form a straight line from your hands to your feet, so the engagement of your abdominals and your gluteus maximus is imperative.

- When first starting out, try adding a small hop to help you lift your feet off the floor if you are having difficulty pressing up.

- To practice proper body alignment, before inverting, try lying on your back flat on the floor with your arms overhead while flexing your abdominals and gluteus maximus as strongly as you can. If done correctly, your lower back should be flat to the floor with no gap.

- Try the same thing lying on your stomach flat on the floor with your arms overhead while flexing your abdominals and gluteus maximus as strongly as you can. If done correctly, your stomach should make no contact with the floor.

GATEWAY POSE:

WIDE LEG FORWARD FOLD

(Prasarita Padottanasana)

Wide leg forward fold is a variation of forward fold with your legs in a straddle position. It opens your hips and hamstrings and is a restorative gentle inversion in its most basic form.

Wide leg forward fold serves as a gateway into deeper forward folds, inversions, and arm balances.

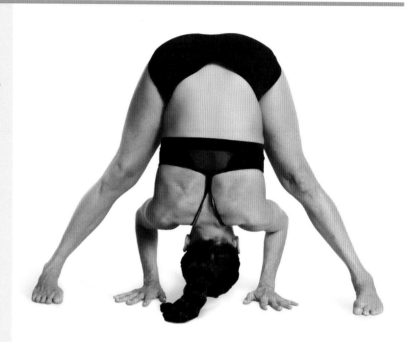

HOW TO GET THERE:

- Begin in a standing position, and step your feet wide into a straddle position.

- Hinge at your waist, fold your upper body forward, and allow your head to hang down toward the floor.

- Place your hands on the floor in front of your face. With your hands on the floor, lift your chest as high as you can to lengthen your spine with a slight bend in your knees if necessary. Fold forward once again, and reach the crown of your head toward the floor.

WHERE TO ENGAGE:

- Draw your navel in and up toward your spine to protect your lower back and create the space to fold deeper.

- Flex your abdominal muscles to help release through your lower back.

- Squeeze through your quadriceps to stretch deeper into your hamstrings.

- Squeeze your elbows in like you would in a chaturanga.

ANATOMY NOTES/ TIPS & TRICKS:

- Shift the weight out of your heels and more onto the balls of your feet to stack your hips over your ankles.

- The tendency is for your toes to want to turn out. Point your toes straight ahead or slightly inward, and roll weight to the outside of your feet as you lift up through your arches.

- Gaze back between your legs to keep your neck long and relaxed.

WIDE LEG FORWARD FOLD ADVANCED ASANA:
HANDS AT WAIST *(Prasarita Padottanasana B)*

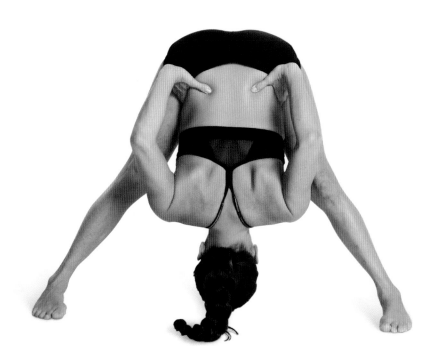

HOW TO GET THERE:

- Begin in a standing position, and step your feet wide into a straddle position.

- Place your hands on your waist with your thumbs wrapped around the back side of your body and four fingers of each hand wrapped around the front side of your body.

- Lift your chest, draw your belly in, and hinge at your waist to fold forward, letting the crown of your head hang down toward the floor.

WHERE TO ENGAGE:

- Draw your navel in and up toward your spine to protect your lower back and create the space to fold deeper.

- Squeeze your hands in at your waist to remind you to engage through your core.

- Squeeze through your quadriceps to stretch deeper into your hamstrings.

ANATOMY NOTES/ TIPS & TRICKS:

- Shift weight out of your heels and more onto the balls of your feet to stack your hips over your ankles.

- The tendency is for your toes to want to turn out. Point your toes straight ahead or slightly inward, and roll weight to the outside of your feet as you lift up through your arches.

- Be active in your arms as you squeeze your waist and draw your elbows back toward one another.

WIDE LEG FORWARD FOLD ADVANCED ASANA:
BINDING SHOULDER OPENER
(Prasarita Padottanasana C)

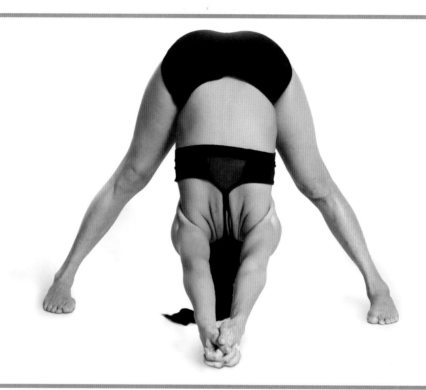

HOW TO GET THERE:

- Begin in a standing position, and step your feet out into a straddle position.

- Interlace your hands together behind your back.

- With your knees slightly bent, hinge at your waist, fold forward, and allow your head to hang down toward the floor. Keeping the bind, reach your arms over your head.

WHERE TO ENGAGE:

- Draw your navel in and up toward your spine to protect your lower back and create the space to fold deeper.

- Keep your palms squeezed in as closely as possible as you reach your arms over your head.

- Squeeze through your quadriceps to stretch deeper into your hamstrings.

ANATOMY NOTES/ TIPS & TRICKS:

- Shift weight out of your heels and more onto the balls of your feet to stack your hips over your ankles.

- The tendency is to want to separate your palms as you fold forward to get your arms farther over your head, but keep them together and touching if possible.

- If your shoulders are too tight to bind, use a towel or a strap.

WIDE LEG FORWARD FOLD ADVANCED ASANA:
BIG TOES *(Prasarita Padottanasana D)*

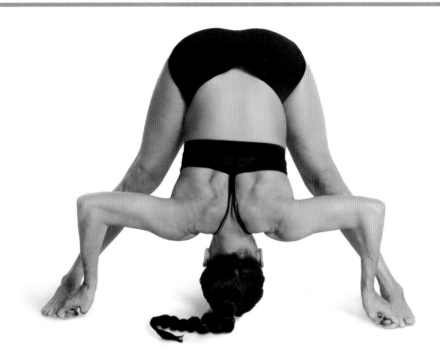

HOW TO GET THERE:

- Begin in a standing position, and step your feet out into a straddle position.

- With your knees slightly bent, hinge at your waist, fold forward, and allow your head to hang down toward the floor.

- Wrap your index and middle fingers around your big toes. While still holding your toes, lift your chest as high as you can to lengthen your spine. Keep your knees slightly bent as you do this. Fold forward once again, and reach the crown of your head toward the floor.

WHERE TO ENGAGE:

- Draw your navel in and up toward your spine to protect your lower back and create the space to fold deeper.

- Flex your abdominal muscles to help release through your lower back.

- Squeeze through your quadriceps to stretch deeper into your hamstrings.

ANATOMY NOTES/ TIPS & TRICKS:

- Shift weight out of your heels and more onto the balls of your feet to stack your hips over your ankles.

- Visualize your hips lifting up as the crown of your head reaches down, and gaze back between your legs to keep your neck long and relaxed.

- The tendency is for your toes to want to turn out. Point your toes straight ahead or slightly inward, and roll weight to the outside of your feet as you lift up through your arches.

- Keep your spine as straight as possible in the fold.

WIDE LEG FORWARD FOLD ARM BALANCE:
FIREFLY *(Titibasana)*

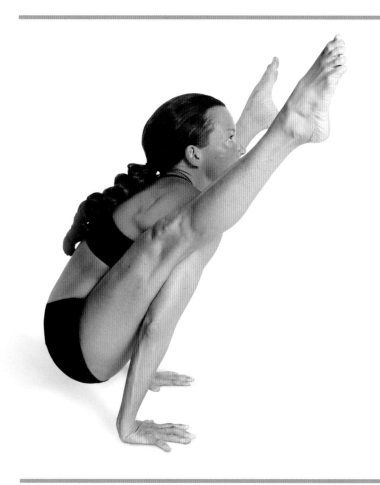

WHERE TO ENGAGE:

- Press strongly into your palms to support your body in the arm balance.

- Squeeze and lift up through your abdominals and pelvic floor.

- Flex your quadriceps to straighten your legs.

ANATOMY NOTES/ TIPS & TRICKS:

- The first step here is to get comfortable sitting with your thighs on your upper arms and balancing. Practice this before you worry about the full expression of the pose.

- Really reach through your chest to help you open into the pose.

- The last step will be fully extending the legs and lifting them up. Depending on the openness of your hips and hamstrings, this might look different for everyone.

HOW TO GET THERE:

- Begin in one of the wide leg forward folds previously listed, and release any bind you may have.

- Bend your knees deeply, and place your palms on the floor behind your heels. Work your arms underneath your legs so that your hamstrings are sitting on top of your triceps.

- Shift your hips back, and bring weight onto your palms to get light in your legs. Bring your feet forward a bit to get leverage and begin to float your toes off the floor.

- Slightly tilt your pelvis forward, straighten your legs, reach through your chest, and take your gaze forward.

WIDE LEG FORWARD FOLD INVERSION:
STRADDLE HEADSTAND

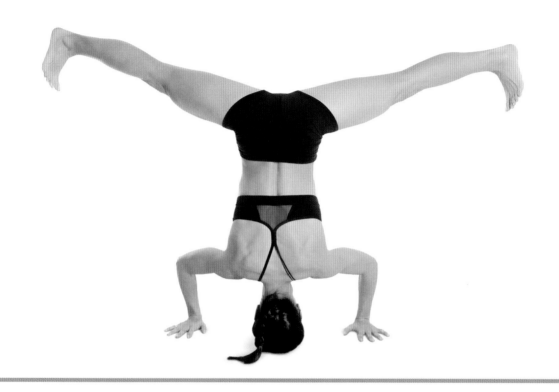

HOW TO GET THERE:

- Begin in wide leg forward fold with your hands under your face.

- Bend your knees, and bring the crown of your head onto the floor and your knees onto your triceps.

- Lift your toes to balance your knees on your triceps and then squeeze through your legs to straighten and lift up into a headstand.

WHERE TO ENGAGE:

- Press into your palms to be sure you are not placing excess stress on your neck and spine. Squeeze your arms in like chaturanga.

- Engage through your core and your legs as you lift into headstand.

- Squeeze your inner thighs in together once you are in the inversion.

ANATOMY NOTES/
TIPS & TRICKS:

- Be sure the crown of your head is directly on the floor and you are not on your forehead.

- Begin by just getting comfortable balancing with your knees on your triceps and your toes lifted off the floor.

- Once you are able to confidently lift into headstand with bent knees, begin to lift up with straight legs without placing your knees on your triceps.

WIDE LEG FORWARD FOLD INVERSION:
STRADDLE HANDSTAND PRESS

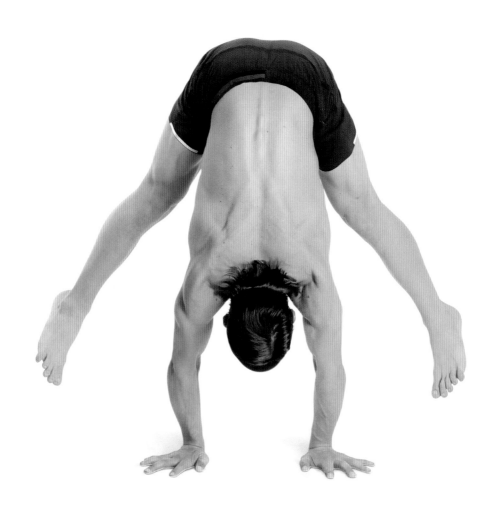

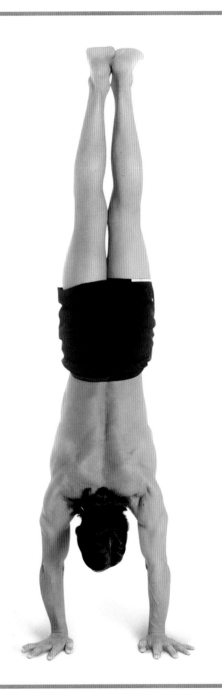

HOW TO GET THERE:

- Begin in one of the variations of wide leg forward fold previously listed and release any bind you may have.

- Lift your gaze, lengthen your spine, and place your hands flat on the floor.

- Keep your gaze lifted, looking between your hands, and coming high onto your toes, while keeping your elbows fully extended and your shoulders externally rotated for stability.

- Shift your weight onto your hands until your toes leave the floor and your hips come slightly in front of your shoulders.

- As you lift your legs upward, your hips will continue to shift even more forward in front of your shoulders until your legs are parallel to the floor.

- Once your legs are above parallel, gradually shift your hips back over your shoulders until they align, and squeeze your thighs together to touch.

WHERE TO ENGAGE:

- Actively flex your abdominal muscles to prevent backward momentum and your gluteus maximus to prevent yourself from folding forward at your waist and coming down.

- Engage your triceps to keep your elbows in full extension.

- Squeeze your inner thighs to keep your legs together.

ANATOMY NOTES/TIPS & TRICKS:

- The goal is to form a straight line from your hands to your feet, so the engagement of your abdominals and your gluteus maximus is imperative.

- When first starting out, try adding a small hop to help you lift your feet off the floor if you are having difficulty pressing up.

GARLAND OR HINDI SQUAT *(Malasana)*

Squatting is one of the most basic functional movements for the human body, but it has become increasingly difficult for many people. As we have evolved into more and more of a sitting culture, many have lost the mobility to deeply squat with proper form. Weak and tight hips, ankles, butts, and hamstrings are the cause for the lack of mobility.

Garland pose, or Hindi squat as some like to call it, is an excellent pose for reclaiming that mobility and also for opening the hips, hamstrings, groin, lower back, and ankles for more advanced asanas.

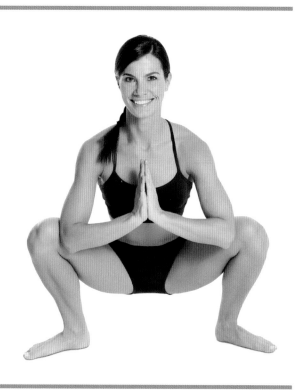

HOW TO GET THERE:

- Place your feet anywhere from hip distance to mat distance apart.

- Bend your knees, and lower your butt down toward the floor.

- Bring your hands to heart center and your elbows to the inside of your knees.

- Lift your chest, straighten your spine as much as possible, and ground down into your feet.

WHERE TO ENGAGE:

- Press your palms together, and press your elbows into your inner thighs.

- Lock in through your pelvic floor, and draw your belly in and up.

ANATOMY NOTES/ TIPS & TRICKS:

- The goal is to eventually squat with your feet under your hips, but take them as wide as necessary to get into the pose and slowly work them in as your body opens more.

- Try to get your heels down to the floor. If they do not touch, fold your mat or roll up a blanket and place it under your heels so that you can relax into the pose.

- If full expression of the pose is too deep, try sitting on a block.

GARLAND POSE ARM BALANCE:
CROW *(Bakasana)*

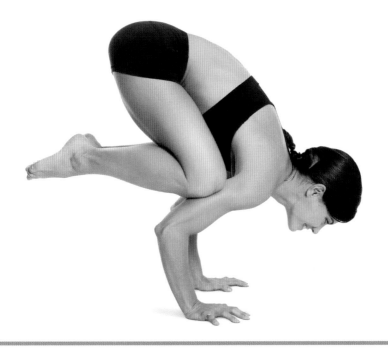

HOW TO GET THERE:

- Begin in garland pose.
- Bring your palms to the floor and your knees to your upper arms.
- Stack your knees on top of your triceps as close to your armpits as possible. Bring your toes together to touch.
- Shift weight forward, and lift your toes off the floor.

WHERE TO ENGAGE:

- Bring a lot of weight forward, and really press into your palms, grip into your fingertips, and lift up through your chest.
- Squeeze your elbows in like you would in a chaturanga, staying very active in your arms.
- Think heels to butt, and really lift up through your legs.
- Draw your abdominal wall in and up to help support the weight of your body in the arm balance.

ANATOMY NOTES/ TIPS & TRICKS:

- Shift more weight forward than you think is necessary, and feel the weight in your palms and fingertips.
- Envision your whole body engaging and lifting up. Nothing should be loose or disengaged here.
- If you are struggling with the arm balance, place your feet on a block and your palms on the floor. This helps get you into the proper position for crow, and you can begin to practice lifting one foot off the block and then two for the arm balance.

GARLAND POSE ARM BALANCE:
SHOULDER PRESSING *(Bhujapidasana)*

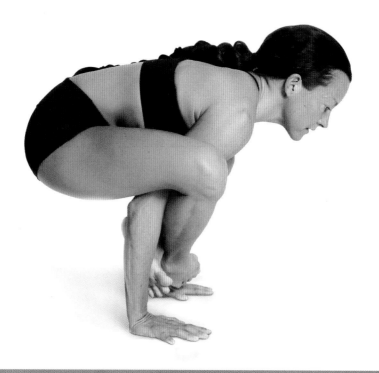

HOW TO GET THERE:

- Begin in garland pose.

- Let your chest come forward a little and your upper back round to bring your palms down to the floor behind your heels.

- Work your arms under your legs so that your thighs are resting on your upper arms.

- Move your feet out in front of you a little more as you sit back onto your palms. Your legs should form a diamond shape.

- Rock your weight back and forth gently to float your feet off the floor.

- Cross your right ankle over your left.

- Lift your chest, and press into your palms to straighten your arms as much as possible.

WHERE TO ENGAGE:

- Press strongly into your palms to support your body in the arm balance.

- Squeeze and lift up through your abdominals and your pelvic floor.

- Flex your toes to your shins and squeeze your ankles together.

- Hug your inner thighs into your outer arms.

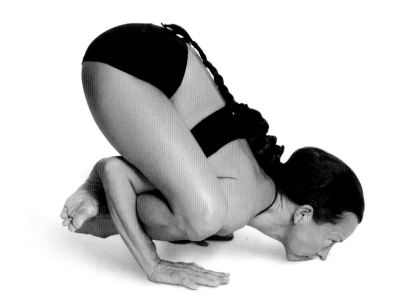

ANATOMY NOTES/ TIPS & TRICKS:

- Place your hands on blocks if you need more space and leverage to balance with your ankles crossed.

- Once you've mastered the first balancing position, move into full expression of the pose by bending your elbows and bringing your chest and chin forward. Your chin will rest on the floor and your heels should shift back behind you.

GARLAND POSE ADVANCED ASANA:
BROKEN WING BIRD

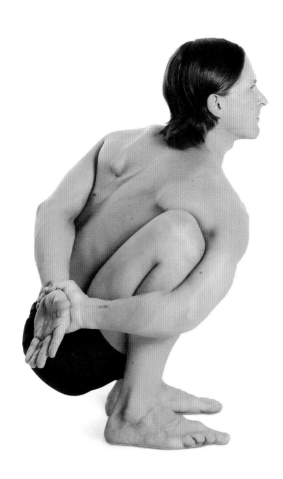

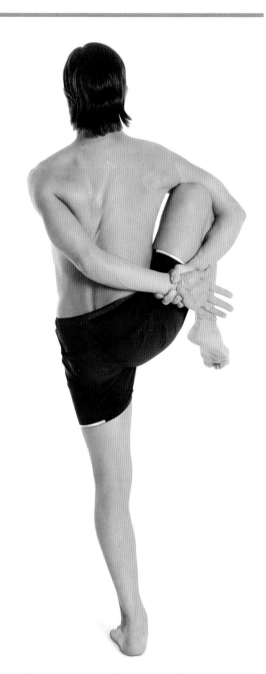

HOW TO GET THERE:

- Begin in garland pose.
- Reach your right hand to the outside of your right toes, internally rotate your upper arm, and bend your elbow to bring your right hand toward your right hip crease.
- Reach your left hand behind your back, and find a bind with your right hand.
- Shift weight onto your left foot, and come high onto your right toes.
- Keep shifting over toward your left, and begin to come to a standing position while maintaining the bind around your right side.
- Straighten the standing leg, and lift your chest.

WHERE TO ENGAGE:

- Tightly wrap your upper arm into your inner thigh to help maintain the bind.
- Squeeze through your left quad to help facilitate the upward lift to standing.

ANATOMY NOTES/ TIPS & TRICKS:

- The hardest part of this pose is finding the bind. Really reach your arm away from you, and then exaggerate the internal rotation to help wrap your arm around your leg.
- Don't try to stand up too fast. Take your time, and really feel the transfer of weight.
- If your shoulders are too tight to bind, use a towel or strap.

GARLAND POSE ARM BALANCE:
BABY CROW

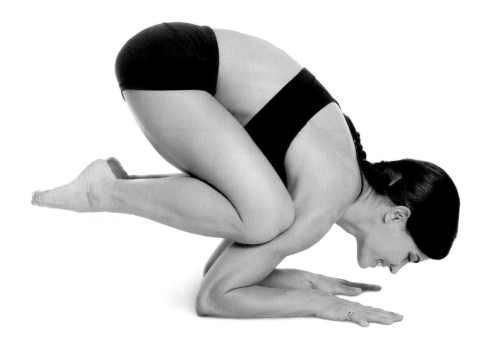

HOW TO GET THERE:

- Begin in garland pose.

- Bring your forearms down to the floor and stack your knees on your upper arms like you do for crow.

- Shift weight forward, and take your gaze to your fingertips.

- Begin to lift one leg up and then two to balance.

WHERE TO ENGAGE:

- Squeeze your knees into your upper arms.

- Squeeze your elbows in like you would in a chaturanga, staying very active in your arms and not letting your elbows come beyond parallel.

- Think heels to butt, and really lift up through your legs.

- Draw your abdominal wall in and up to help support the weight of your body in the arm balance.

ANATOMY NOTES/ TIPS & TRICKS:

- Shift more weight forward than you think is necessary, and feel the weight in your forearms, palms, and fingertips.

- Envision your whole body engaging and lifting up. Nothing should be loose or disengaged here.

- Baby crow is deceptively harder than crow pose because your center of gravity is so close to the floor. This pose will build shoulder and core strength.

GATEWAY POSE:

WHEEL *(Urdhva Dhanurasana)*

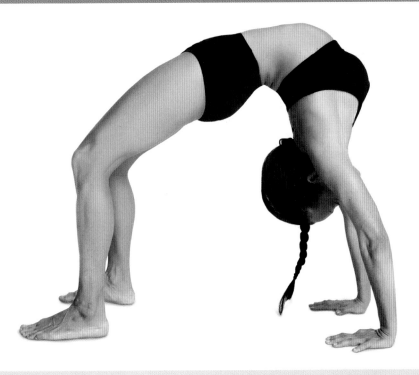

Backbending postures are included in virtually every yoga practice. They are beneficial for heart opening and stimulation of the nervous system. Many beginning practitioners are surprised to learn that backbends are actually one of the healthiest things you can do for the spine. Both forward and back bending promote circulation to the vertebrae, keeping them healthy and mobile.

Wheel is one of the more common backbends practiced in yoga, and many students mark the ability to perform this pose as a milestone in their practice. It's a demanding posture that requires a combination of both flexibility and strength.

Practicing wheel develops strength in the many areas of the body, including wrists, upper back, shoulders, and thighs. It also stretches the chest, abdomen, and upper back.

Once you can comfortably perform full expression of wheel, begin to incorporate these variations into your practice.

(continued on next page)

GATEWAY POSE:

WHEEL *(continued)*

HOW TO GET THERE:

- Begin by lying down on your mat with your knees bent and your feet hip distance apart.

- Bend your elbows, and place your hands behind your shoulders with your palms on the floor and your fingertips facing your shoulders.

- Press into your hands and feet, and lift your hips up toward the ceiling as you reach your chest toward the back of the mat.

- Fully extend your arms, and bring your shoulders to stack over your wrists.

WHERE TO ENGAGE:

- Root down through all four corners of your feet, and stay strong in your legs.

- Reach your chest through your shoulders, and focus on opening and lengthening through the front side of your body.

ANATOMY NOTES/ TIPS & TRICKS:

- Focus on drawing your tailbone down and toward your knees to ensure you don't compress your spine.

- Even if you're not able to fully extend your arms and stack your shoulders over your wrists, you are still experiencing tons of benefits from the backbend. To help get deeper into your spine, try coming onto the balls of your feet and lifting your heels off the mat, or place blocks against a wall shoulder-width apart, horizontal and flat. Place your hands on the blocks in same position as wheel pose with your fingers hanging off the edge.

- One of the most common mistakes you could make is to lose the engagement of your legs. Prevent this is by placing a block between your thighs and squeezing as you perform the pose.

WHEEL ADVANCED ASANA:
INVERTED STAFF POSE
(Dwi Pada Viparita Dandasana)

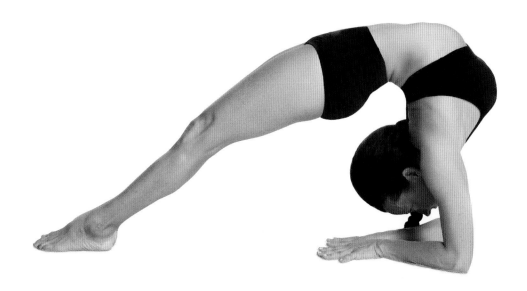

HOW TO GET THERE:

- Begin in forearm variation of backbend.
- Walk your feet toward the top of the mat as much as you need to bring your feet together and your big toes to touch.
- Straighten your legs.

WHERE TO ENGAGE:

- Press down through the entire length of your forearms, and reach your chest through your shoulders.
- Keep your thighs spiraling in toward one another
- Ground down through the base of your big toes.

ANATOMY NOTES/ TIPS & TRICKS:

- If any excessive pressure is felt in your lower back, try widening your stance.

WHEEL ADVANCED ASANA:
DROP BACK

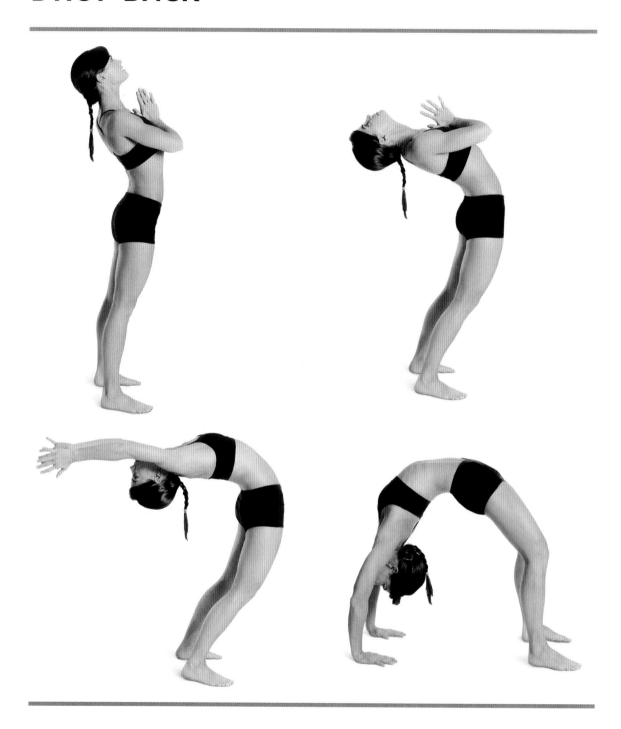

HOW TO GET THERE:

- Begin in a standing position with your feet placed directly under your hips. Bring your hands to heart center.

- Lift your chin and chest up until your gaze is toward the ceiling.

- As your head falls back and you continue to extend your spine into an inverted C-shape, counter by allowing your hips to move forward.

- Once you can see the floor behind you, reach your hands down toward the mat until your arms are fully extended, and then bring your palms down, coming into wheel pose.

WHERE TO ENGAGE:

- Press into all four corners of your feet, and stay strong in your legs.

ANATOMY NOTES/ TIPS & TRICKS:

- It's normal to feel fear and apprehension when first attempting drop backs. To help alleviate this, use a spotter or practice the pose with the assistance of a wall. Place your feet one arm's-distance away from the wall. Once you get to the point where your head falls back, place your hands against the wall with your palms flat and your fingers facing the floor. Walk your hands down to the floor.

- Once you get comfortable dropping back, try coming back up to standing. Begin by rocking back and forth to transfer weight more onto your legs. Build some momentum with the rocking until you can lift your hands from the floor and come to stand. Your head is the last thing to lift. Bringing it up too early can cause a loss of balance.

WHEEL ADVANCED ASANA:
FOREARMS

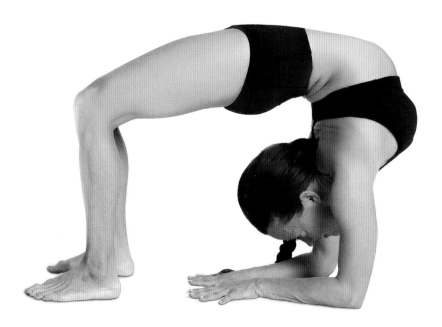

HOW TO GET THERE:

- Begin in wheel.

- Bend your elbows and drop down to the crown of your head.

- Supporting the weight of your head with one arm, bring your opposite forearm down to the floor, followed by your other forearm.

- Bring your palms close enough together to interlace your fingers.

WHERE TO ENGAGE:

- Press down through the entire length of your forearms, and reach your chest through your shoulders.

- Press into your feet, and stay strong in your legs.

ANATOMY NOTES/ TIPS & TRICKS:

- Focus on drawing your tailbone down and toward your knees to ensure you don't compress your spine.

- To exit this backbend, drop the crown of your head to the floor, place both of your hands on the floor next to your head, and press back into wheel.

2

Standing Poses

In this section, we explore how routine standing postures such as warrior one, side angle, and half moon can take you into a variety of different inversions, arm balances, and advanced asanas.

These common postures feature a host of uncommon variations that do everything from challenging balance and strength to opening your body in new and different ways.

GATEWAY POSE:

WARRIOR ONE *(Virabhadrasana I)*

Warrior one is perhaps the most commonly known of the standing asanas. Yoga classes from nearly every lineage utilize this posture. It's the key pose in sun salutations and is often used to heat and warm the body. This energizing posture stretches the hips, belly, groin, and chest and opens the lungs and rib cage.

The variations of warrior one that we explore here range from shoulder and hip opening options to arm balances.

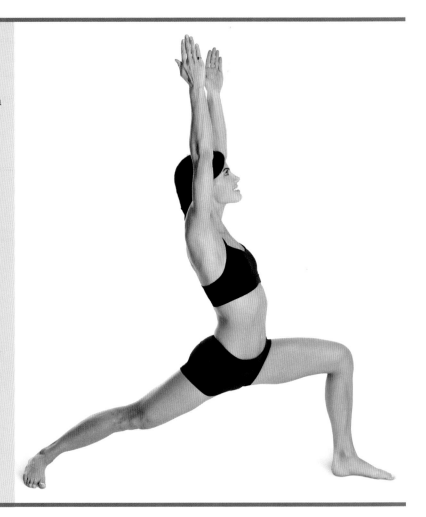

HOW TO GET THERE:

- Begin in down dog. Step your left foot between your hands, and drop your back heel flat to the floor.

- Keep your front knee bent so that your left thigh is parallel to the mat, and lift your arms up overhead.

WHERE TO ENGAGE:

- Press through the blade of your back foot to keep your arch lifted.

- Engage your right inner thigh to help rotate your hips forward.

ANATOMY NOTES/ TIPS & TRICKS:

- Keep your front knee stacked directly over your ankle.

- If your knee is moving past your ankle, lengthen your stance.

- Keep your shoulders relaxed away from your ears and your tailbone dropping down.

WARRIOR ONE ADVANCED ASANA:
HUMBLE WARRIOR *(Baddha Virabhadrasana)*

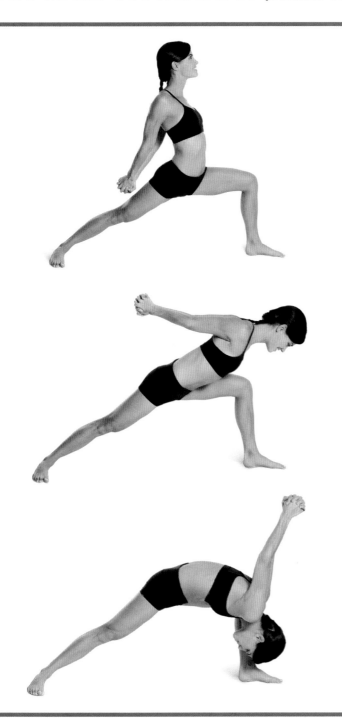

HOW TO GET THERE:

- Begin in warrior one on the left side.

- Interlace your fingers together behind your back with your palms flat.

- Keep your elbows straight, and hinge at your waist to fold forward.

- Allow your head to hang and your hands to reach overhead.

WHERE TO ENGAGE:

- Press through the blade of your back foot to keep your arch lifted.

- Keep lifting through your right inner thigh.

- Actively press your hands together overhead toward the floor.

- Engage abdominal muscles to release through your lower back, and fold deeper toward the floor.

ANATOMY NOTES/ TIPS & TRICKS:

- Notice if your hips are swaying to the left, and realign them toward the midline of your body to keep them square.

- If your shoulders are too tight to bind, use a towel or a strap.

WARRIOR ONE ARM BALANCE:
FLYING SPLITS *(Eka Pada Koundinyasana II)*

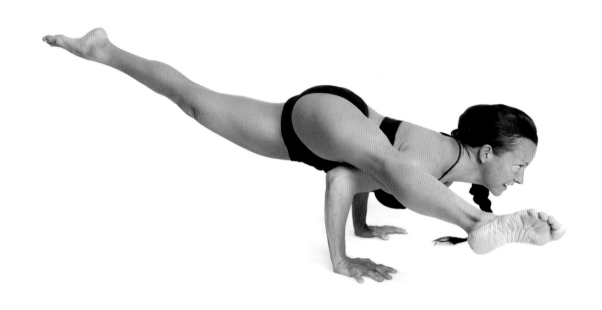

HOW TO GET THERE:

- Begin in humble warrior on the right side, and release your hands down to the floor with your palms flat.

- Work your right shoulder underneath your right thigh, bringing your thigh as high onto your tricep as possible.

- Shift your gaze forward, and come high onto the ball of your back foot.

- Keep your elbows bent, and start to shift weight forward onto your hands. Extend your right foot straight out in front of you, and let your left foot float off the mat.

WHERE TO ENGAGE:

- Firmly press your fingertips into the mat.

- Engage the hamstring and gluteus of your back leg to lift it up.

- Squeeze the quadriceps of your front leg to straighten it.

- Reach your chest forward.

ANATOMY NOTES/ TIPS & TRICKS:

- Just because you can't do full splits doesn't mean you can't do this posture. A helpful modification is to walk your foot over to the right side of the mat so that as your foot lifts, it's at an angle instead of straight forward.

- If your hamstrings are open enough for full splits, a key to keeping your toes straight forward is to roll your inner thigh up your arm toward your shoulder.

WARRIOR ONE ADVANCED ASANA:
BIRD OF PARADISE *(Svarga-Dvijasana)*

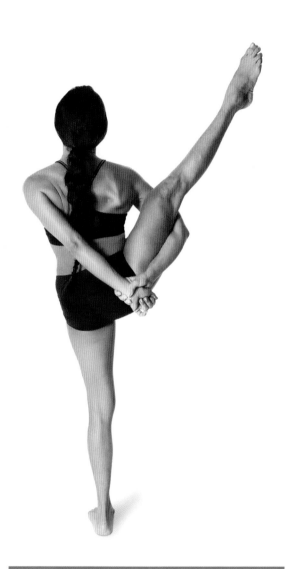

HOW TO GET THERE:

- Begin in humble warrior on the right side, and release your hands down to the floor with your palms flat.

- Start with your right arm, internally rotate your right shoulder as you drop it underneath your right thigh, and reach your right hand behind your back with your palm facing up.

- Reach your left hand behind your back, grasping your fingers together or, if you have the space, wrapping your right hand around your left wrist.

- Once your bind is secure, look forward and shift weight onto your right foot. Step your left foot up until it's parallel with your right.

- Keep your left knee bent, and transfer weight onto your left leg, coming high onto the ball of your right foot.

- Slowly rise to stand, straightening your left leg. Once you feel balanced, extend your right leg straight up.

WHERE TO ENGAGE:

- The standing leg is your foundation. Press down firmly to stand tall.

- Lift your chest, and pull your shoulders back.

- Squeeze the quadriceps of your right leg to lengthen your hamstring.

ANATOMY NOTES/TIPS & TRICKS:

- The key to success in this posture is to ensure you have a stable foundation. The standing leg should be completely straight before you attempt to straighten the lifted leg.

WARRIOR ONE ARM BALANCE:
SCISSORS *(Astavakrasana)*

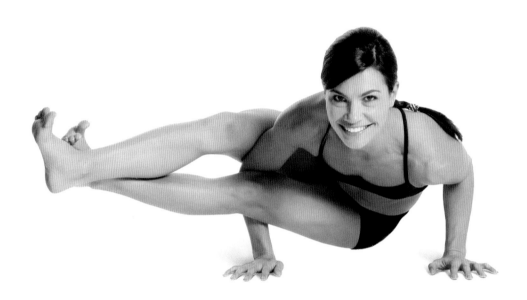

HOW TO GET THERE:

- Begin in flying splits.

- Flex your spine, lift your upper back toward the ceiling, and draw your left knee into your chest. Straighten your arms as much as you need to get your knee to your chest, and keep your left toes pointed.

- Thread your left foot to the outside of your right wrist and cross your left ankle over your right.

WHERE TO ENGAGE:

- Press against the floor with your fingertips.

- Engage your abdominal wall, drawing in and up.

- Once you come into scissors, squeeze your inner thighs into your arms and reach through your heels.

ANATOMY NOTES/ TIPS & TRICKS:

- The transition from flying splits to scissors can be tricky, but break it down by first getting comfortable drawing your back knee into your chest. You may have to really press into your palms and straighten through your arms to create the clearance to thread your left leg through for scissors.

- Keep your chest and hips parallel to the floor. Squeezing your inner thighs together will facilitate this.

- Scissors is not a posture about strength. Keeping your shoulders stacked over your wrists will provide all the support you need in your arms. The strong engagement of your legs is the most vital part.

GATEWAY POSE:
SIDE ANGLE *(Parsvakonasana)*

Side angle provides a stretch through the side body while also opening and lengthening the groin, chest, and spine. Practicing this pose builds strength in the legs and ankles.

One of the most common variations of side angle is a bind behind the back that opens the shoulders. We explain how to get into this bind and all of the exciting places you can go once you've secured it. Learn how to perform the commonly taught bird of paradise pose, binding half moon, and more.

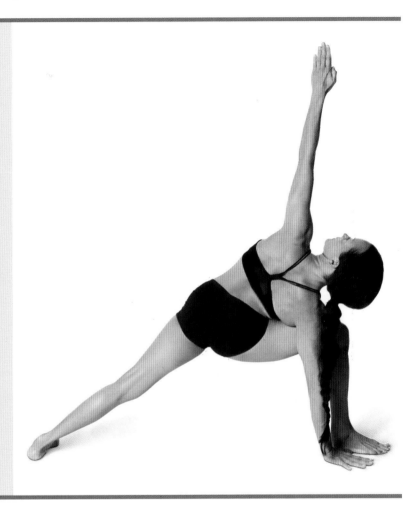

HOW TO GET THERE:

- Begin in down dog. Step your right foot between your hands and drop your back heel flat to the floor.

- Keep your front knee bent so that your right thigh is parallel to the mat.

- Keep your right hand down to the inside of your right shin, and lift your left hand straight up.

WHERE TO ENGAGE:

- Press through the blade of your back foot to keep your arch lifted.

- Press your right upper arm and right shin together to keep your knee aligned over your ankle and open your chest.

ANATOMY NOTES/ TIPS & TRICKS:

- Keep your front knee stacked directly over your ankle.

- If your knee is moving past your ankle, lengthen your stance.

SIDE ANGLE ADVANCED ASANA:
BOUND SIDE ANGLE (Baddha Utthita Parsvakonasana)

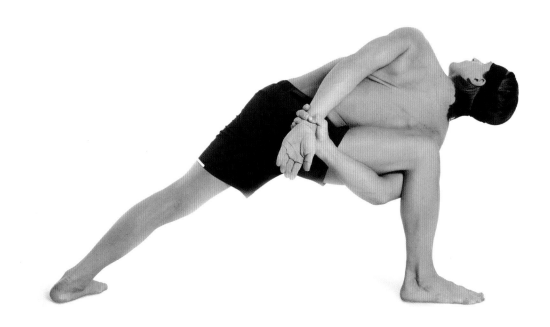

HOW TO GET THERE:

- Begin in side angle.

- Gaze down toward your right hand, and drop your chest below your right thigh. Internally rotate your right shoulder, and reach your right hand behind your back with your palm facing up.

- Look up to open your chest, and reach your left hand behind your back. Interlace your fingers together, or wrap your right hand around your left wrist to find the bind.

WHERE TO ENGAGE:

- Press through the blade of your back foot to keep your arch lifted.

ANATOMY NOTES/ TIPS & TRICKS:

- If makes it easier, internally rotate your shoulders to get into the bind. It's almost like you're collapsing your posture down. Once you've achieved the bind, engage back into the posture by externally rotating your shoulders and opening your chest.

- Use a towel or strap if you need assistance with the bind.

SIDE ANGLE ADVANCED ASANA:
BIRD OF PARADISE *(Svarga-Dvijasana)*

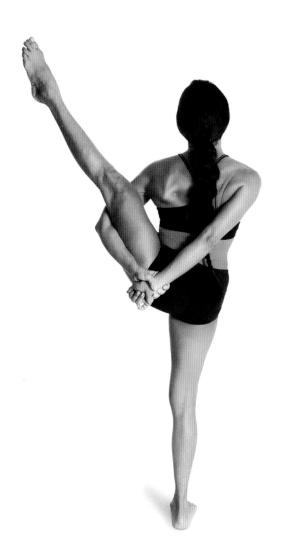

HOW TO GET THERE:

- Begin in bound side angle on the left side.

- Once your bind is secure, look forward, and shift your weight onto your left foot. Step your right foot up until it's parallel with your left.

- Keep your right knee bent, transfer weight onto your right leg, and come high onto the ball of your left foot.

- Slowly rise to stand, straightening your right leg. Once you feel balanced, extend your left leg straight up.

WHERE TO ENGAGE:

- The standing leg is your foundation. Press down firmly to stand tall.

- Lift your chest, and pull your shoulders back.

- Squeeze the quadriceps of your right leg to lengthen your hamstring.

ANATOMY NOTES/TIPS & TRICKS:

- The key to success in this posture is to ensure you have a stable foundation. The standing leg should be completely straight before attempting to straighten the lifted leg.

- Once you can confidently perform bird of paradise, try to hinge at your waist and fold forward. Your chest should be parallel to the mat and your toes facing forward. Hold for a few breaths, and slowly lift back into bird.

SIDE ANGLE ADVANCED ASANA:
BINDING HALF MOON *(Baddha Ardha Chandrasana)*

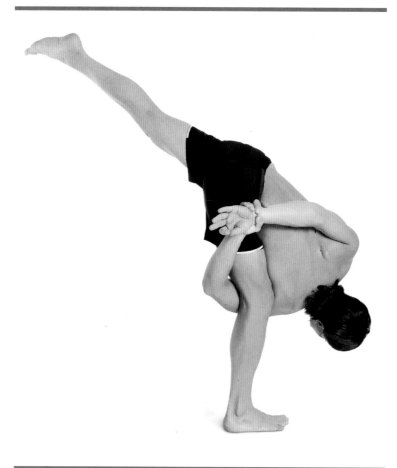

HOW TO GET THERE:

- Begin in bound side angle on the right side.

- Once your bind is secure, gaze down toward the floor, soften your right knee, and shift weight onto your right foot.

- Shift your chest forward in front of your right foot until you feel your left foot leave the ground.

- Balancing on your right leg, lift your left leg parallel to the mat as you pull your toes to your shin and reach through your heel.

WHERE TO ENGAGE:

- Engage through your outer left thigh to lift it parallel to the floor.

ANATOMY NOTES/
TIPS & TRICKS:

- Keeping your gaze to the floor is a good way to maintain stability in this pose. As you feel more confident in the pose, try lifting your gaze and rotating your chest upward.

- Keeping your right knee bent is another way to maintain stability in this pose. As you feel more confident in the pose, try straightening the standing leg.

SIDE ANGLE ADVANCED ASANA
VISVAMITRA'S POSE *(Visvamitrasana)*

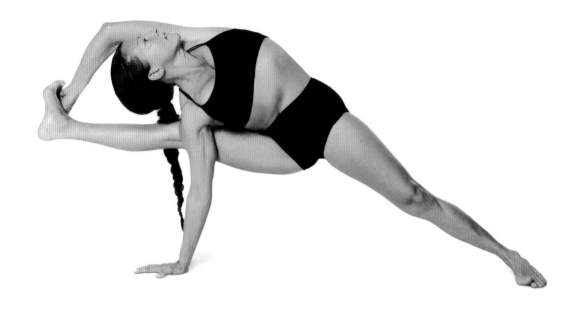

HOW TO GET THERE:

- Begin in side angle on the right side.

- Look down and begin to lower your chest toward the floor so that it's below your right thigh.

- Move your right palm under and to the outside of your right thigh.

- Lift your gaze, and begin to shift weight onto your right hand. As you straighten your right arm, walk your right foot into the middle of the mat until it leaves the ground.

- Weight is completely balanced on your right arm and back leg. Your left hand takes the outside blade of your right foot. Tuck your chin, and begin to rotate your torso up toward the ceiling. At the same time, work to straighten through your right leg.

- Once your right leg and right arm are completely extended, tilt your head back and gaze up.

WHERE TO ENGAGE:

- Engage your tricep to fully extend your right arm.

- Press firmly through your back foot to keep your arch lifted.

- Engage your quadriceps to straighten your right leg, and reach through your heel to find more length.

ANATOMY NOTES/ TIPS & TRICKS:

- Keep your shoulder directly over your elbow and your elbow directly over your wrist to make the workload easier on your arm and allow you to focus more on the opening in the left side of your body and hamstring.

- For a modified variation of Visvamitrasana, drop down to your left knee, and untuck your toes before you begin transitioning into this pose.

GATEWAY POSE:

HALF MOON *(Ardha Chandrasana)*

Half moon is an exciting pose that tests balance and concentration. Once you become comfortable balancing in half moon, you can begin to explore how expansive and powerful this pose can be. Deep side body opening, backbending, and difficult balance challenges are available through different variations of the posture.

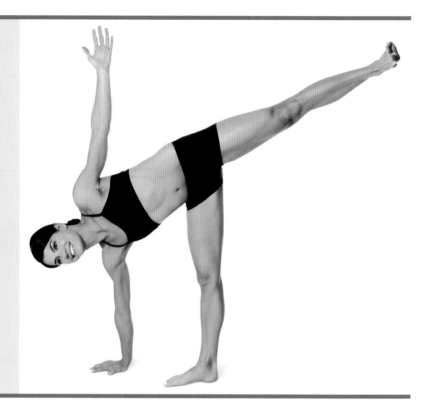

HOW TO GET THERE:

- Begin in down dog. Step your right foot between your hands.

- Keep both palms flat to the mat, and shift your weight onto your right leg until your left leg is parallel with the mat and the standing leg is straight. Keep your hips square.

- Keep your right palm down 6 to 8 inches (15 to 20 cm) in front of your right foot, and reach your left hand up toward the ceiling.

- As you rotate your chest open, stack your left hip on top of your right, and reach through the heel of your left foot.

- Once you feel stable, lift your gaze toward your left hand.

WHERE TO ENGAGE:

- Press down firmly through the standing leg.

- Flex through the quadriceps of the lifted leg to extend the leg long.

- Engage your outer left thigh to keep your leg parallel to the floor.

ANATOMY NOTES/ TIPS & TRICKS:

- Your right hand on the floor is a secondary source of support. The standing leg should make up the majority of your foundation.

- This posture is best experienced when you can stack your hips. If your right hamstring is too tight to allow for this, come high onto your right fingertips, or use a block under your right hand.

HALF MOON ADVANCED ASANA:
BALANCING HALF MOON

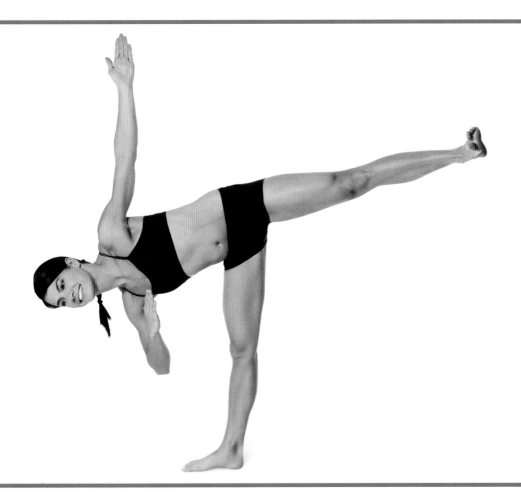

HOW TO GET THERE:

- Begin in half moon on the right side.

- Once you feel stable in the posture, bring your right hand to heart center.

WHERE TO ENGAGE:

- Press down firmly through the standing leg.

- Flex through the quadriceps of the lifted leg to extend the leg long.

- Engage your outer left thigh to keep your leg parallel to the floor.

ANATOMY NOTES/ TIPS & TRICKS:

- If you're having trouble balancing, take your gaze down to the floor for added stability. Softening your right knee will add similar support.

- For an added challenge, bring your left hand to meet your right at heart center.

HALF MOON ADVANCED ASANA:
HALF BOW BOUND HALF MOON
(Ardha Chandra Chapasana)

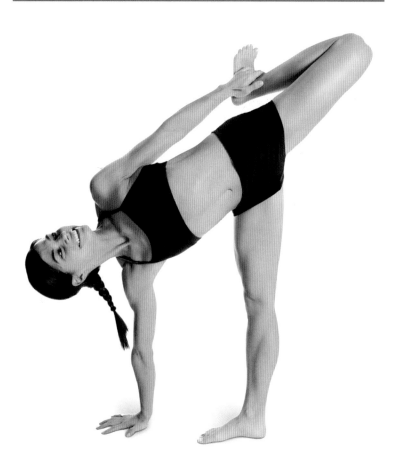

HOW TO GET THERE:

- Begin in half moon on the right side.

- Bend your left knee, and reach your left hand for your left ankle.

- Kick your hand and foot away from your body into a half bow, open your chest, and let your head fall back.

WHERE TO ENGAGE:

- Press down firmly through the standing leg.

- Fire through your left quadriceps to get deeper into the backbend.

ANATOMY NOTES/ TIPS & TRICKS:

- The more you kick your hand and foot together, the more it will be necessary to counter this by shifting your hips in the opposite direction.

- You can also experience a quadriceps stretch in this pose by pulling your heel in toward your glutes instead of kicking it away.

HALF MOON ADVANCED ASANA:
CARTWHEEL

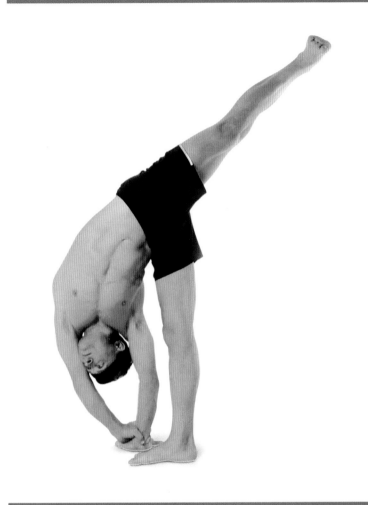

HOW TO GET THERE:

- Begin in half moon on the right side.

- Bring your gaze down to the mat, and reach your left hand over your head toward the mat.

- Shift weight forward, lift your left leg higher, and place your left palm flat to the floor with your fingertips facing your foot, or wrap your left hand around your right wrist.

WHERE TO ENGAGE:

- Press down firmly through the standing leg.

- Flex through the quadriceps of the lifted leg to extend the leg long.

ANATOMY NOTES/ TIPS & TRICKS:

- Lifting your left leg above parallel while your left hand reaches down is what gives this posture the illusion of moving into a cartwheel.

- To take this pose deeper, slide your right palm into alignment with your right heel, and turn your fingertips toward the right side of the mat. Tuck your chin, and wrap your left hand around your right wrist. Pull your chest through your shoulders, and rotate the right side of your chest upward. Tilt your head back.

HALF MOON ADVANCED ASANA:
DOUBLE BOUND HALF MOON
(Funky Chapasana)

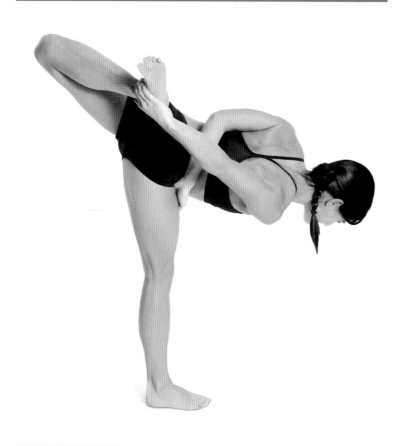

HOW TO GET THERE:

- Begin in half moon on the right side.

- Keep your gaze lifted, and reach your left hand behind your back to the crease of your right hip.

- Keeping all the weight on your right leg, bend your left knee, and reach your right hand back for your left ankle.

- Once bound, kick your foot and hand away from your body, and press your hips in the opposite direction.

WHERE TO ENGAGE:

- Press down firmly through the standing leg.

- Fire through your left quadriceps to get deeper into the backbend.

ANATOMY NOTES/ TIPS & TRICKS:

- The key to this posture is to continue to lean back into the backbend and not to break at your waist. Resist the temptation to look down.

- Soften your right knee if you need more stability.

GATEWAY POSE:

REVOLVED HALF MOON

(Parivrtta Ardha Chandrasana)

Give your half moon a twist with the revolved variation. Revolved half moon stretches the hips and hamstrings while also strengthening the legs and providing a deep twist.

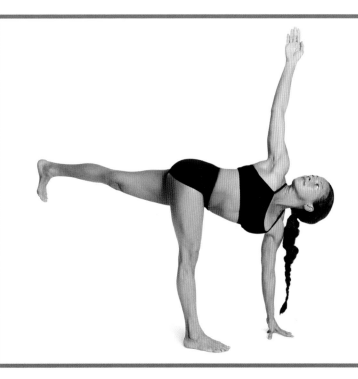

HOW TO GET THERE:

- Begin in downward facing dog. Step your right foot between your hands.

- Keep both palms flat to the mat, and shift your weight into your right leg until your left leg is parallel with the mat and the standing leg is straight. Keep your hips square.

- Keep your left palm down next to your right foot, and reach your right hand up toward the ceiling.

- Rotate from your waist up along the axis of your spine until your right shoulder is stacked over your left. Your right palm opens to the right.

- Lengthen your spine, and lift your gaze upward.

WHERE TO ENGAGE:

- Flex through the quadriceps of your back leg to fully extend.

- Engage abdominals and obliques to achieve the rotation of your torso.

- Press through the standing leg to keep your hips square.

ANATOMY NOTES/ TIPS & TRICKS:

- Squaring your hips is the most important aspect of this posture. If your hamstrings are tight and preventing you from achieving this, try softening the standing leg or using a block under the hand that's grounded.

- The most common compensation students make is allowing the extended leg to drop down and sway off-center in the direction they are rotating. Try practicing this posture with the extended leg pressing into a wall to ensure square hips.

REVOLVED HALF MOON ADVANCED ASANA:
ONE LEG BIND

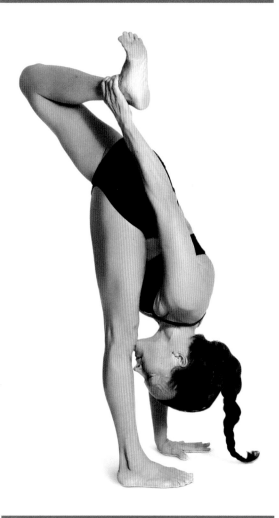

HOW TO GET THERE:

- Begin in revolved half moon on the right side.

- Gaze down to the floor, bend your left leg, and reach your right hand for your left ankle.

- Fold your forehead to your shin, and reach your left knee toward the ceiling.

- Square your hips.

WHERE TO ENGAGE:

- Flex your left hamstring to pull your left heel toward your gluteus, and release through your quad.

- Engage abdominals to fold forward, and release through your lower back.

- Engage the right quadriceps to release the right hamstring.

ANATOMY NOTES/TIPS & TRICKS:

- This posture is going to provide a big stretch for the quadriceps. The flexibility of the quadriceps will determine how much you can square your hips while lifting your knee upward.

- The most common compensation students make is allowing the extended leg to drop down and sway off-center in the direction they are rotating. Try practicing this posture with the extended leg pressing into a wall to ensure square hips.

REVOLVED HALF MOON ADVANCED ASANA:
REVOLVED DANCER *(Parivrtta Natarajasana)*

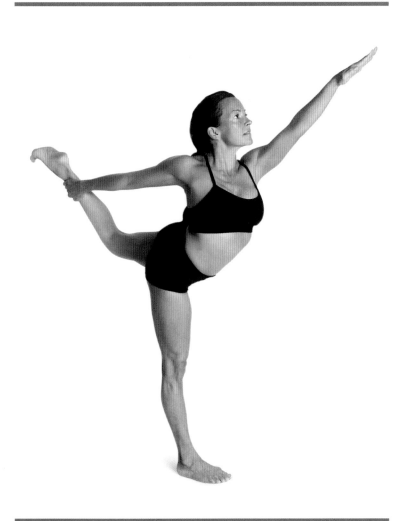

HOW TO GET THERE:

- Begin in revolved half moon on the right side.

- Gaze down to the floor, bend your left leg, and reach your right hand for your left ankle.

- Soften the standing leg, lift your gaze, and slowly rise to standing.

- Only when you feel stable, begin to straighten the standing leg, and kick your hand and foot into one another.

- Keep your chest and gaze lifted and your hips square to the floor.

WHERE TO ENGAGE:

- Engage the right quadriceps to extend the standing leg.

- Press your left foot into your right hand to open into the backbend.

ANATOMY NOTES/ TIPS & TRICKS:

- Balance is the greatest obstacle, both as you come from the floor to standing and extending into your fullest expression of the posture. Take your time with the transitions.

- Wait until you are completely upright to begin kicking your hand and foot together into the backbend position.

GATEWAY POSE:

TRIANGLE *(Trikonasana)*

Triangle is a feel-good standing pose. With two grounded and straight legs, you can really focus on stretching and expansion in this pose without the added element of breathing into a bent leg or balancing. Triangle features a multitude of benefits, including stretching and strengthening both the upper body and lower body while also providing stress relief and improved digestion.

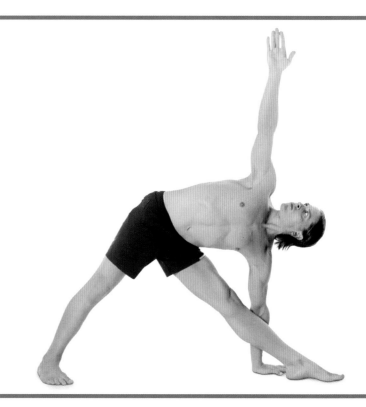

HOW TO GET THERE:

- Begin in down dog. Step your right foot between your hands, and drop your back heel flat to the floor.

- Straighten your right leg, and place your right hand to the inside or outside of your right foot with your palm flat.

- Reach your left hand up, rotating the right side of your chest up toward the ceiling until your spine is fully extended.

- Stack your left hip on top of your right.

- Lift your gaze upward.

WHERE TO ENGAGE:

- Press through your right big toe and the outside blade of your left foot to keep your left arch lifted.

- Engage the right quadriceps to lengthen the hamstring.

- Squeeze your left gluteus to help stack your left hip on top of your right.

ANATOMY NOTES/ TIPS & TRICKS:

- If looking upward bothers your neck, look straight ahead.

- Straightening both legs is the most important aspect of this posture. If your hamstrings are too tight to allow you to straighten both legs while keeping your palm flat on the floor, try using a block under your grounded hand or placing your hand on your shin.

TRIANGLE ADVANCED ASANA:
STAR SIDE PLANK *(Vasisthasana)*

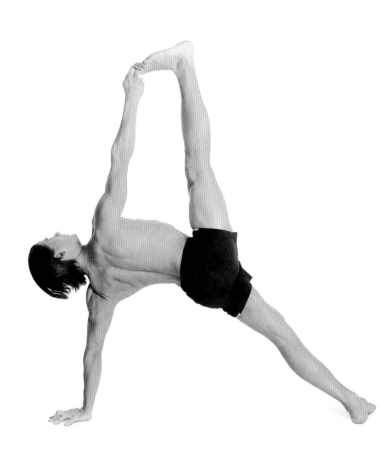

HOW TO GET THERE:

- Begin in triangle on the right side. Look down and hook your right index and middle fingers around your right big toe.

- Place your left palm flat on the floor, coming high onto the ball of your back foot.

- Simultaneously roll to the outside of your left heel, and begin to reach your right leg up toward the ceiling.

- Pull your right toes back and reach through your heel. Feel the right side of your body lift upward.

WHERE TO ENGAGE:

- Press firmly into your grounded palm to stabilize through your shoulder.

- Squeeze through the quadriceps of your extended leg to lengthen the hamstring and straighten your leg.

ANATOMY NOTES/ TIPS & TRICKS:

- Gaze up toward the lifted leg.

- Make sure you feel your fingertips pressing down into the mat to prevent placing all the weight in your palm and compressing your wrist.

- For an extra core challenge, release your toes, and let your extended leg hover in the star position.

TRIANGLE ADVANCED ASANA:
BOUND TRIANGLE *(Baddha Trikonasana)*

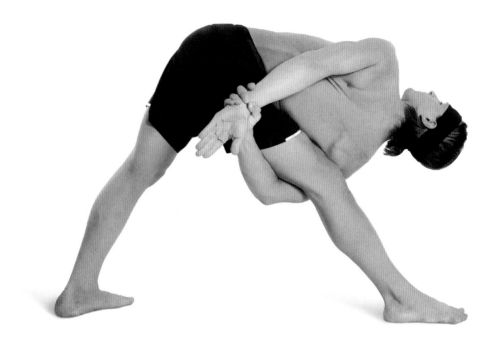

HOW TO GET THERE:

- Begin in triangle on the right side.

- Gaze down toward the floor, and soften your right knee.

- Reach your right hand under your right thigh and behind your back.

- Direct your gaze back up, and reach your right hand behind your back.

- Interlace your fingers together, or wrap your right hand around your left wrist to find the bind.

WHERE TO ENGAGE:

- Press through the blade of your back foot to keep your arch lifted.

- Engage the right quadriceps to straighten your right leg.

ANATOMY NOTES/ TIPS & TRICKS:

- Bound triangle is easier if you internally rotate your shoulders to get into the bind, almost like you're collapsing your posture down. Once you've achieved the bind, engage back into the posture by externally rotating your shoulders and opening your chest.

- Use a towel or strap if you need assistance with the bind.

GATEWAY POSE:

CRESCENT LUNGE *(Anjaneyasana)*

Crescent lunge, or high lunge as it's commonly called, is a combination lunge and backbend. The lunge portion of the pose strengthens the butt and quadriceps while stretching the hip flexor. The backbend in the upper body opens the thoracic spine, chest, and lungs.

Crescent lunge leads you into deep twists, challenging balancing variations, and arm balances.

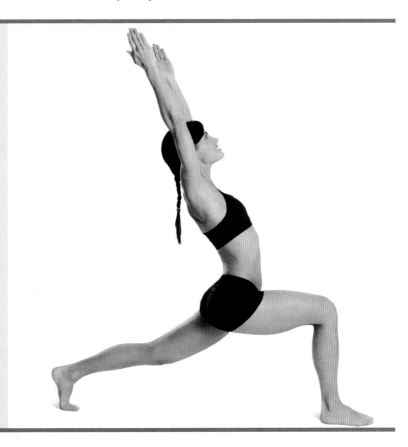

HOW TO GET THERE:

- Begin in down dog. Lunge your right foot between your hands, and stay high on the ball of your back foot.

- Rise to standing, and reach your arms overhead.

- Keep your right thigh parallel to the mat, and push through the heel of your left foot to straighten your leg.

WHERE TO ENGAGE:

- Engage your left quad to extend your left leg straight.

- Utilizing the transverse abdominis, draw your navel in and up to extend your spine and protect your lower back.

- Engage your left gluteus to release through your left hip flexor.

ANATOMY NOTES/ TIPS & TRICKS:

- Keep your front knee stacked directly over your ankle.

- If your knee is moving past your ankle, lengthen your stance.

- Keep your shoulders relaxed away from your ears and your tailbone dropping down.

- A stretch should be felt through your left quad and hip flexor with no compression of your lower back.

- Your pelvis should be pointing straight forward. If it's angling down, soften your back knee to create better alignment.

CRESCENT LUNGE ADVANCED ASANA:
PRAYER TWIST *(Parivrtta Anjaneyasana)*

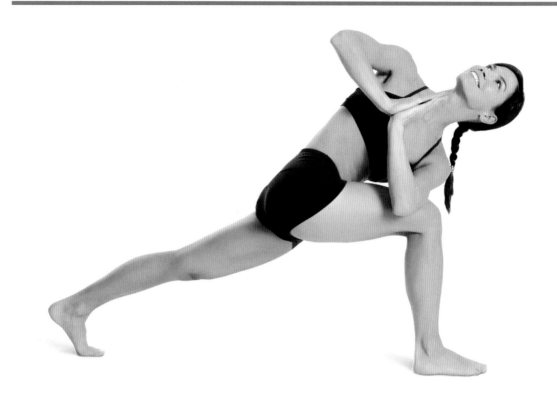

HOW TO GET THERE:

- Begin in crescent lunge on the right side.

- Bring your hands to prayer position at heart center.

- Twist your left elbow to the outside of your right knee.

- Once your elbow is secure, fully extend your spine while rotating the left side of your chest, and gaze upward.

WHERE TO ENGAGE:

- Draw your navel in and upward to engage the transverse abdominals. This creates space to twist.

- Abdominals and obliques are responsible for the rotation of your spine into the twist.

- Engage through your left quad to keep you stable and secure as you twist.

- Use your left arm pressing into your right thigh as leverage to deepen the twist.

ANATOMY NOTES/ TIPS & TRICKS:

- The most important aspect of this posture is the twist. If your balance is unstable as you twist, ground your left knee down to the floor.

CRESCENT LUNGE ARM BALNCE:
SIDE CROW SPLITS

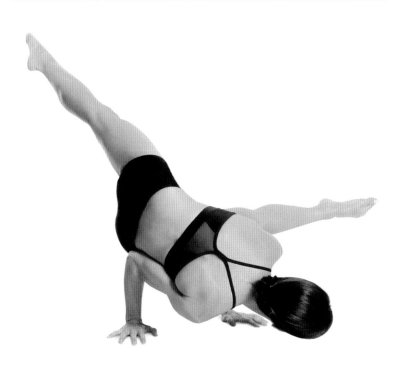

WHERE TO ENGAGE:

- Stay active in your fingertips to prevent placing all of the weight into your palms and compressing your wrists.

- Squeeze your elbows in, and keep them in line with your shoulders to maintain a base of support.

- Squeeze through the quadriceps of both legs to straighten them.

ANATOMY NOTES/ TIPS & TRICKS:

- This posture isn't about strength but rather alignment. As long as your elbows stack over your wrist at a 90-degree angle, your body will feel light.

- Visualize your hips lifting so you don't collapse your weight downward into your arms.

- Gaze forward or to the side.

- Prayer twist is a great gateway to side crow splits because your body is perfectly aligned for the arm balance. Trust yourself to lean into it and go for it.

HOW TO GET THERE:

- Begin in crescent lunge prayer twist on the right side.

- Soften your back knee, and gaze at the floor on the outside of your right thigh. Place your palms flat on the floor on the outside of your right leg.

- Start to bend your elbows, and lean weight into your arms. Rest your right thigh on top of your left tricep.

- Keep bending your elbows to 90 degrees, and allow the weight of your body to be fully supported by your arms.

- Extend both legs straight.

CRESCENT LUNGE ADVANCED ASANA:
BOUND CRESCENT TWIST
(Baddha Parivrtta Anjaneyasana)

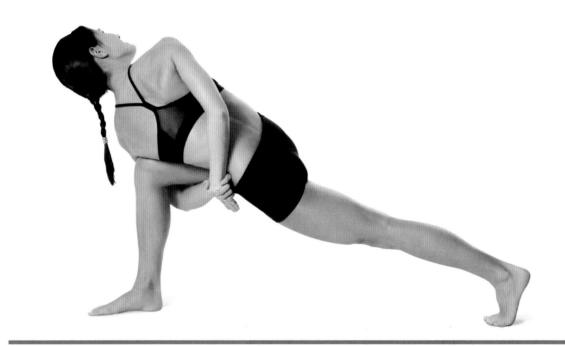

HOW TO GET THERE:

- Begin in prayer twist on the right side.

- Gaze down to the floor, and reach your left hand under your right thigh and behind your back.

- Reach your right hand behind your back and either interlace your fingers or wrap your left hand around your right wrist to secure the bind.

- Lift your gaze back up, and lean back to rotate your chest open and fully extend your spine.

WHERE TO ENGAGE:

- Draw your navel in and upward to engage the transverse abdominis. This creates more space to twist.

- Abdominals and obliques are responsible for the rotation of your spine into the twist.

- Engage through your left quad to keep you stable and secure as you twist.

ANATOMY NOTES/ TIPS & TRICKS:

- Internally rotate your left shoulder to help you find the bind. Once you've achieved the bind, engage back into the posture by externally rotating your shoulder and opening your chest.

- If you are having difficulty binding, try dropping your knee to bind. If you feel stable, tuck your toes; re-straighten your left knee, and lift it off the ground.

- If shoulders are too tight to bind, use a towel or strap to assist with the bind.

CRESCENT LUNGE ADVANCED ASANA:
BOUND REVOLVED HALF MOON
(Baddha Parivrtta Ardha Chandrasana)

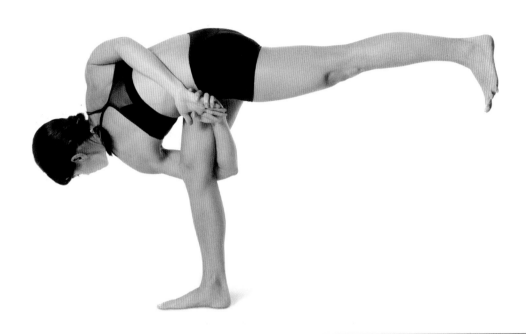

HOW TO GET THERE:

- Begin in bound crescent twist on the right side.

- Gaze down to the floor in front of your right foot.

- Maintaining your bind, soften your back knee, and shift weight onto your right leg.

- Lift your left leg off the ground. Once your leg is parallel to the mat and your left hip is square with your right, begin to straighten your right leg.

WHERE TO ENGAGE:

- Engage both quadriceps to straighten your legs.

- Keep the transverse abdominis drawn in for support and stability.

ANATOMY NOTES/ TIPS & TRICKS:

- The important aspect of this posture is maintaining a bind as you balance on the standing leg. Keeping your right knee soft will assist with balance. As you feel more stable, straighten the standing leg.

- Keeping your gaze down also helps with balance. As you feel ready, move your gaze straight ahead or upward. When you lift your gaze, extend your spine.

CRESCENT LUNGE ADVANCED ASANA:
REVOLVED BIRD OF PARADISE
(Parivrtta Svarga-Dvijasana)

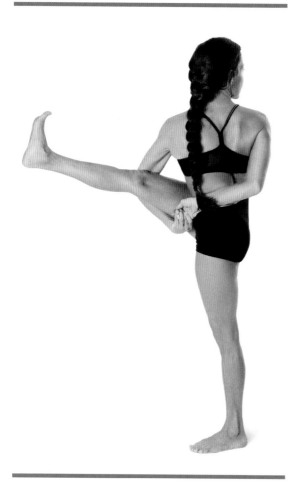

HOW TO GET THERE:

- Begin in bound crescent twist on the right side.

- Gaze down to your right foot, and step your left foot up to meet your right.

- Maintaining your bind, soften your left knee, and shift weight into your left leg.

- Slowly rise to a standing position, keeping your right knee bent.

- Once you come to a full standing position with your left leg straight and you feel balanced, extend your right leg out straight, rotate your chest open, and pull your shoulders back.

WHERE TO ENGAGE:

- Engage both quadriceps to straighten your legs once you're in a full standing position.

- Draw your belly in and up to provide stability and space to twist deeper.

ANATOMY NOTES/TIPS & TRICKS:

- The important aspect of this posture is maintaining a bind as you balance on the standing leg. Keeping your left knee soft will assist with balance. As you feel more stable, straighten the standing leg.

- Your biggest key to success with this pose is to know when you feel confident about the steps it takes to get there. Be slow and intentional about moving into this posture.

GATEWAY POSE:

STANDING SPLITS *(Urdhva Prasarita Eka Padasana)*

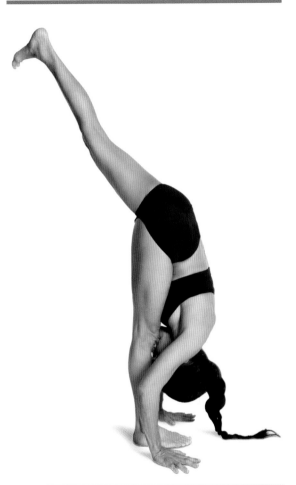

HOW TO GET THERE:

- Begin in down dog. Lunge your right leg between your hands, and shift weight forward onto your right leg.

- Lift your left leg up, and fold your forehead in toward your right shin.

- Straighten both legs.

WHERE TO ENGAGE:

- Engage the quadriceps to straighten both legs.

- Draw the transverse abdominis in and up to create space for the forward fold and to take it deeper.

ANATOMY NOTES/TIPS & TRICKS:

- Standing splits is a deep hamstring opener. A straight lifted leg is more important than a straight grounded leg. If your hamstrings are tight, keep your knee soft on the grounded leg, reducing the intensity of the stretch.

- Point your left toes down toward the floor, and keep your hips square. Resist the urge to open your hips in order to get your lifted leg higher.

Standing splits is a simple pose that provides an excellent way to stretch and lengthen the hamstrings while also serving as a gentle, calming inversion. Standing splits are one of the best poses for transitioning into handstand.

STANDING SPLITS ADVANCED ASANA:
ARROW/BALANCING

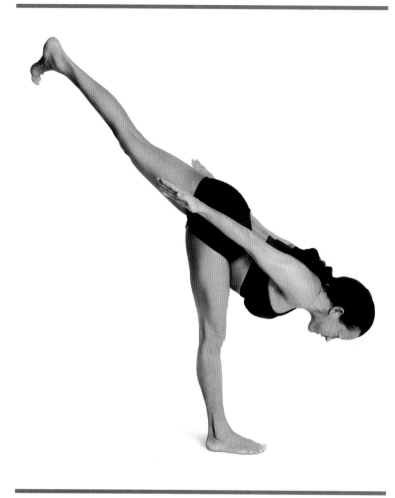

HOW TO GET THERE:

- Begin in standing splits on the right side.

- Gaze forward in front of your right foot. Lift your chest slightly off your thighs to create a straight line from your head to your heel.

- Slowly extend both arms straight back behind you with fingertips, reaching toward the extended leg and turning the palms in.

WHERE TO ENGAGE:

- Engage the quadriceps to straighten both legs.

- Reach through your fingertips toward your extended leg as you lift up through your chest.

ANATOMY NOTES/
TIPS & TRICKS:

- This pose is a huge balance challenge. Work your way into it slowly. Start by bringing your hands to heart center, and get comfortable balancing there before extending them all the way back.

- Soften your knee on the standing leg to help with balance.

STANDING SPLITS INVERSION:
HANDSTAND *(Adho Mukha Vrksasana)*

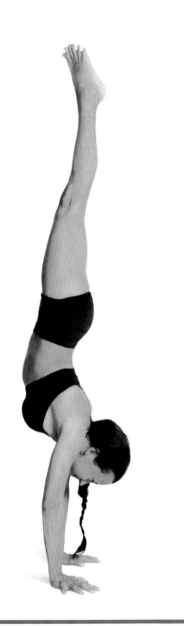

HOW TO GET THERE:

- Begin in standing splits on the right side.

- With both palms flat on the floor, gaze forward in front of your right foot, and lift your chest slightly off your thigh to lengthen your spine.

- Shift weight onto the ball of your right foot, and begin to take some small hops, lifting your left leg toward the ceiling and allowing your right toes to leave the mat.

- Once you find a balance point where your hips stack over your shoulders, bring your right leg up to meet your left.

WHERE TO ENGAGE:

- The lift and engagement of your left leg is crucial for getting into handstand position.

- Actively flex your abdominal muscles to prevent backward momentum and your gluteus maximus to prevent yourself from folding forward at your waist and coming down.

- Engage the triceps to keep your elbows in full extension.

- Squeeze your inner thighs to keep your legs together.

ANATOMY NOTES/TIPS & TRICKS:

- The goal is to form a straight line from your hands to your feet, so the engagement of abdominals and your gluteus maximus is imperative.

- The tendency here is to want to use force to kick up into the handstand. Use body awareness and control instead. The key to lifting into the handstand is getting your hips stacked over your shoulders. Practice taking small hops and really lifting through your left leg to get into this position. Once your hips are over your shoulders, lifting up to handstand is simple.

3

BALANCING POSES

Balancing poses in yoga practice provide both physical and mental benefits. From a physical standpoint, these postures build stability in the body from the floor up and help to strengthen the feet, ankles, knees, and hips. From a mental standpoint, they build focus and confidence.

You can take the physical and mental challenge a step further by exploring variations of balancing postures that take you into arm balances, inversions, and more intense balancing.

EAGLE *(Garudasana)*

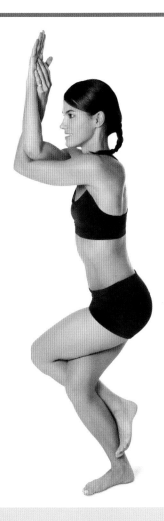

Eagle requires you to balance on one leg while maintaining a bind with your arms that opens your shoulders. This pose can lead you into several varieties of side crow as well as a headstand.

HOW TO GET THERE:

- Begin in a standing position at the top of the mat. Bend your knees slightly.

- Standing on your right leg, pick up your left leg and wrap it up and over your right. Tuck the top of your left foot behind your right calf if you are able.

- Bring your arms out into a T-shape, and then wrap your left arm under your right and rotate your palms together to touch. Lift your elbows up to shoulder height, and press your hands away from your face.

WHERE TO ENGAGE:

- Squeeze your inner thighs together to keep the bind of your legs.

- Engage your abdominals, and keep your chest lifted.

- Press your palms together, and lift up through your fingertips to stretch your shoulders and maintain the arm bind.

ANATOMY NOTES/TIPS & TRICKS:

- Don't worry if you can't get your foot completely wrapped around your calf muscle. Do the best you can.

- If tightness in your shoulders prevents you from achieving the arm bind, bring your hands to prayer position at heart center.

- Keep your torso upright. Your shoulders should stack over your hips.

EAGLE ARM BALANCE:
SIDE CROW *(Parsva Bakasana)*

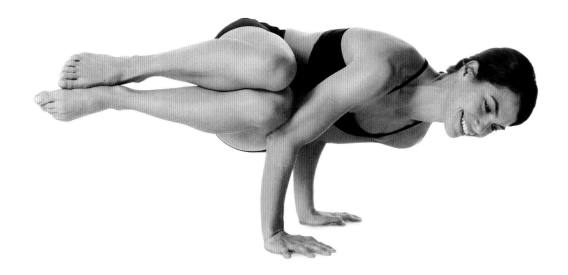

HOW TO GET THERE:

- Begin in eagle on the right side. Release your arm bind.

- Come all the way down into a squatting position on your right toes, and bring your hands to the outside of your left thigh, facing away from you and directly under your shoulders.

- Keep your elbows squeezing in, and bend them to 90 degrees. Allow your left thigh to rest on the shelf created by your arms.

- Bring your right knee on top of your left.

WHERE TO ENGAGE:

- Stay active in your fingertips to prevent placing all of your weight onto your palms and compressing your wrists.

- Squeeze your elbows in, and keep them in line with your shoulders to maintain a base of support.

- Squeeze your inner thighs together and your heels toward your butt.

ANATOMY NOTES/ TIPS & TRICKS:

- This posture isn't about strength but rather alignment. As long as your elbows stack over your wrist at a 90-degree angle, your body will feel light.

- Visualize your hips lifting so you don't collapse your weight downward into your arms.

- Gaze forward or to the side.

EAGLE ARM BALANCE:
SIDE CROW SPLITS

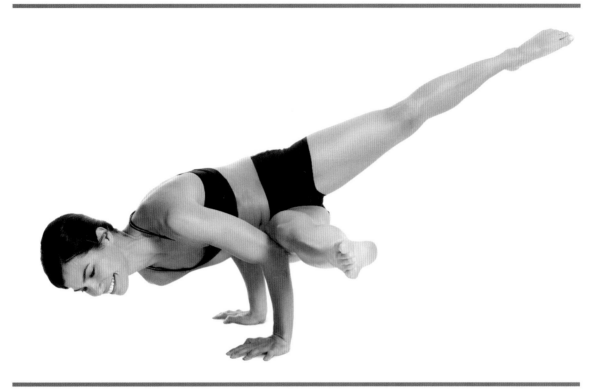

HOW TO GET THERE:

- Begin in eagle on the right side. Release your arm bind.

- Come all the way down into a squatting position on your right toes, and bring your hands to the outside of your left thigh, facing away from you and directly under your shoulders.

- Start to bend your elbows, and lean weight into your arms. Rest your left thigh on top of your right tricep.

- Keep bending your elbows to 90 degrees, and allow the weight of your body to be fully supported by your arms.

- Extend both legs straight by kicking them away from one another.

WHERE TO ENGAGE:

- Stay active in your fingertips to prevent placing all of your weight onto your palms and compressing your wrists.

- Squeeze your elbows in, and keep them in line with your shoulders to maintain a base of support.

- Squeeze through the quadriceps of both legs to straighten them.

ANATOMY NOTES/
TIPS & TRICKS:

- This posture isn't about strength but rather alignment. As long as your elbows stack over your wrist at a 90-degree angle, your body will feel light.

- Visualize your hips lifting so you don't collapse your weight downward into your arms.

- Gaze forward or to the side.

EAGLE ARM BALANCE:
SIDE CROW STRAIGHT LEGS

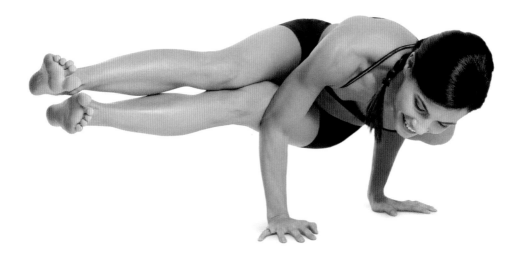

HOW TO GET THERE:

- Begin in eagle. Release your arm bind.

- Come all the way down into a squatting position on your right toes, and bring your hands to the outside of your left thigh, facing away from you and directly under your shoulders.

- Keep your elbows squeezing in, and bend them to 90 degrees. Allow your left thigh to rest on the shelf created by your arms.

- Bring your right knee on top of your left, and extend both legs out straight.

WHERE TO ENGAGE:

- Stay active in your fingertips to prevent placing all of your weight onto your palms and compressing your wrists.

- Squeeze your elbows in, and keep them in line with your shoulders to maintain a base of support.

- Squeeze through the quadriceps to straighten your legs, and reach through your heels.

- Reach your chest forward.

ANATOMY NOTES/ TIPS & TRICKS:

- This posture isn't about strength but rather alignment. As long as your elbows stack over your wrists at a 90-degree angle, your body will feel light.

- Visualize your hips and chest lifting so you don't collapse your weight downward into your arms.

- Gaze forward or to the side.

EAGLE INVERSION:
HEADSTAND WITH EAGLE LEGS

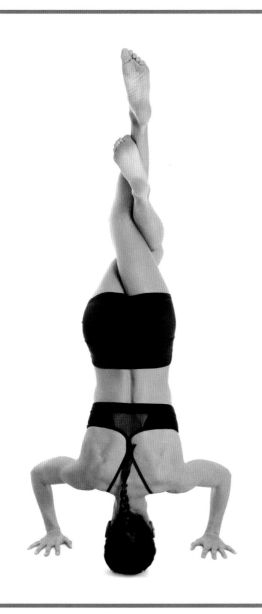

HOW TO GET THERE:

- Begin in eagle.

- Keeping your eagle legs, come down to a squatting position, and place your palms flat on the floor.

- Tuck your chin and place the crown of your head on the floor. Squeeze your elbows in line with your shoulders.

- Still keeping your eagle legs, slowly lift into a headstand.

WHERE TO ENGAGE:

- Squeeze your inner thighs together.

- Abdominals and obliques should be kept active throughout.

ANATOMY NOTES/TIPS & TRICKS:

- Form an equilateral triangle between your hands and head. This means that the distance between your hands should match the distance between either hand and your head, just like a tripod.

- Keep the weight of this pose equally distributed between your head and hands for the greatest sense of stability.

- Your chin should be in a neutral position to ensure your neck is in alignment.

- In order for your legs to lift off the mat, your hips must move forward in front of your shoulders to counter their weight. This requires extremely strong abdominal control and is perhaps the most difficult aspect of this pose.

- To come out of the inversion, hinge at your waist and bring your legs back down to the floor. Slowly rise to stand back in eagle.

- If you're ready to try a more advanced variation, try switching your legs in the air by unwinding them and wrapping your right over your left. Return to standing in eagle on the other side.

GATEWAY POSE:

FIGURE FOUR *(Eka Pada Utkatasana)*

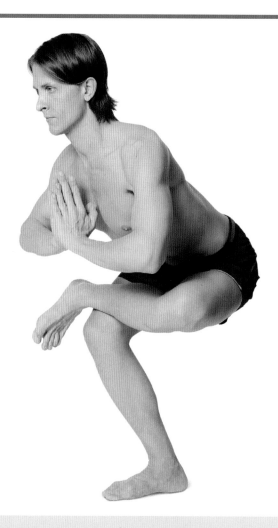

HOW TO GET THERE:

- Begin in a standing position at the top of the mat with your hands at heart center.

- Pick up your left leg and cross your left ankle over your right knee.

- Bend your right knee and squat down. Send your hips back as you reach your chest forward to lengthen your spine.

WHERE TO ENGAGE:

- Press your left knee down toward the floor to open and stretch your left hip and gluteus.

- Reach through your left heel, and pull your toes back toward your shin.

- Keep your abdominals engaged.

ANATOMY NOTES/ TIPS & TRICKS:

- Sink your hips down so that your right thigh is parallel with the mat. Imagine you are sitting back into a chair.

- Extend through the crown of your head, and lengthen your spine. Avoid rounding through your back.

Figure four is a standing hip-opening pose that tests balance and concentration. Once you feel stable in figure four, bring your hands to the floor for an arm balance or inversion.

FIGURE FOUR ARM BALANCE:
FLYING PIGEON *(Eka Pada Galavasana)*

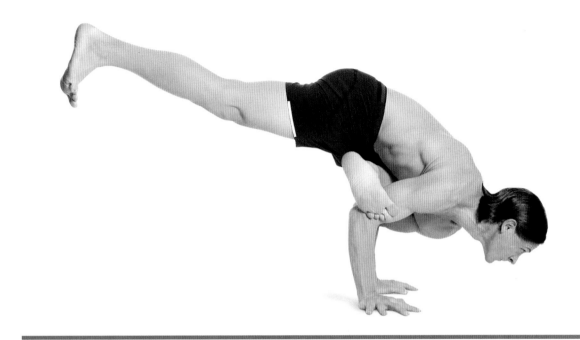

HOW TO GET THERE:

- Begin in figure four on the right side.
- Squat down and place your palms flat on the floor.
- Hook your left toes around your right tricep, and rest your left knee on your left tricep.
- Lean forward and bring weight onto your fingertips. Lift your right toes off the ground.
- Keep your chest lifted, and straighten your right leg behind you.

WHERE TO ENGAGE:

- Flex your left foot to maintain the hook of your toes around your right tricep.
- Lift through your chest, and squeeze in and up through your abdominals.
- Engage your right quadriceps to extend and straighten your leg behind you.
- Stay active in your fingertips to prevent placing all of your weight onto your palms and compressing your wrists.
- Squeeze your elbows in, and keep them in line with your shoulders to maintain a base of support.

ANATOMY NOTES/ TIPS & TRICKS:

- Get comfortable balancing with your right toes off the floor before you attempt to extend and straighten your leg behind you.
- Once you are ready to extend your leg behind you, be mindful to keep everything engaged, squeezing in and lifting up.
- Keep reaching your chest forward and bringing weight into your fingertips to counteract your leg extending back behind you.

FIGURE FOUR ARM BALANCE:
GRASSHOPPER *(Parivrtta Eka Pada Ukatasana)*

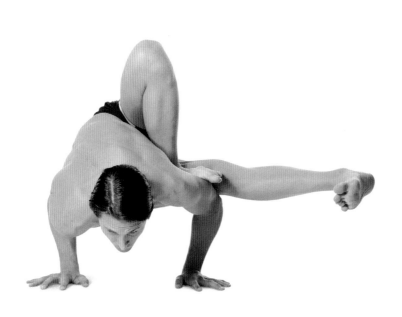

- Stay active in your fingertips to prevent placing all of your weight onto your palms and compressing your wrists.

- Squeeze your elbows in and keep them in line with your shoulders to maintain a base of support.

- Engage your right quadriceps to extend and straighten your leg.

ANATOMY NOTES/ TIPS & TRICKS:

- This pose requires a little bit of everything, with deep twisting, deep hip opening, and arm balancing. Be sure to prep for this pose with figure four and the flying pigeon arm balance.

- You must be able to get your tricep to the sole of your foot in order to attempt the arm balance. If you can't get there, keep practicing the twist until you can.

- Get comfortable balancing with your right heel tucked to your gluteus before you attempt to extend and straighten your leg out to the side.

- If you find that your left foot keeps sliding off your left tricep, try working it closer up toward your armpit, and really press your foot down into your arm to create a shelf.

HOW TO GET THERE:

- Begin in figure four standing on your right leg.

- Twisting deeply, bring your left tricep to the sole of your left foot.

- Squat down and place your hands on the right side of the mat, reaching away from you.

- Look down to the right, and squat down into your right leg. Place your hands shoulder-distance apart on the mat with your fingertips facing away from you.

- Lean into your arms until you are at a 90-degree bend at your elbows and your left foot can rest flat in a standing position on your left tricep.

- Keep your right knee bent with your heel tucked into your gluteus or extend it straight out for full expression of the pose.

WHERE TO ENGAGE:

- This pose requires extremely intense twisting. Draw your navel in and twist deeply from your ribcage. Press your tricep firmly into your foot to deepen the twist.

FIGURE FOUR INVERSION:
HEADSTAND WITH FIGURE FOUR LEGS
(Eka Pada Salamba Shirshasana)

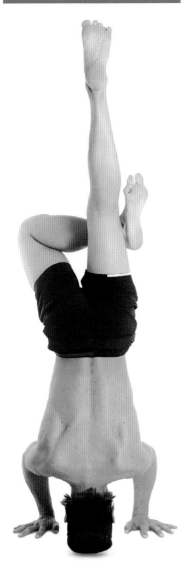

HOW TO GET THERE:

- Begin in figure four or flying pigeon arm balance.

- Keeping your figure four legs, come down to a squatting position, and place your palms flat on the floor.

- Tuck your chin and place the crown of your head on the floor. Squeeze your elbows in line with your shoulders, and flex your left toes into your right tricep.

- Unhook your toes from your triceps, and slowly lift into a headstand as you keep your legs in figure four position.

WHERE TO ENGAGE:

- Flex both feet, and pull your toes back toward your shins.

- Squeeze your quadriceps and inner thighs to stay active in your legs.

- Abdominals and obliques should be kept engaged throughout.

ANATOMY NOTES/ TIPS & TRICKS:

- Form an equilateral triangle between your hands and head. This means that the distance between your hands should match the distance between either hand and your head, just like a tripod.

- Keep the weight of this pose equally distributed between your head and hands for the greatest feeling of stability.

- Your chin should be in a neutral position to ensure your neck is in alignment.

- To come out of the inversion, hinge at your waist, and slowly bring your legs down toward the floor. Re-hook your left toes around your right tricep, and rest your left knee on your left tricep. Transfer weight back into your fingertips, and come back into figure four or flying pigeon arm balance.

- If you're ready to try a more advanced variation, try switching your legs in the air by uncrossing them and then crossing your right ankle over your left. Exit the inversion, and return to figure four or flying pigeon arm balance on the opposite side.

GATEWAY POSE:

DANCER *(Natarajasana)*

Dancer is a balancing pose, featuring a beautiful backbend. It's a powerhouse pose that trains concentration, stretches the hips, chest, and shoulders, and strengthens the feet, ankles, hips, and back of the body.

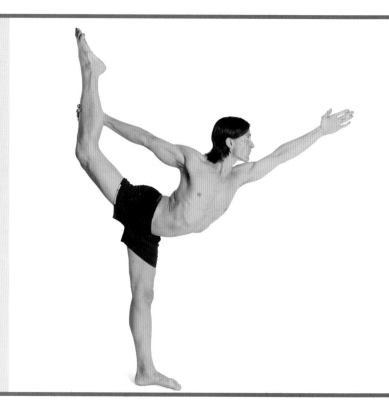

HOW TO GET THERE:

- Begin in a standing position at the top of the mat.
- Reach your right arm straight up with your bicep by your ear.
- Shift weight onto your right leg, and soften your right knee.
- Bend your left knee, and bring your foot up toward your butt.
- Wrap your right hand around the inside of your left foot.
- Kick your hand and foot together, lean forward slightly, and lift through your chest.
- Straighten the standing leg.

WHERE TO ENGAGE:

- Press your hand and foot together to move into the backbend.
- Lift up through your left heel, chest, and right arm.
- Squeeze your right quadriceps to straighten the standing leg.
- Ground down into all four corners of your right foot.

ANATOMY NOTES/ TIPS & TRICKS:

- Keep your hips square to the mat, and avoid rotating your left hip higher than your right just to lift your leg higher.
- The tendency here is to lean forward and forget about the upward lift. Everything should be lifting up toward the ceiling.
- Avoid looking at the floor. Gaze straight out in front of you or up toward your lifted hand.
- Keep your toes pointing straight forward.

DANCER ADVANCED ASANA:
KING DANCER

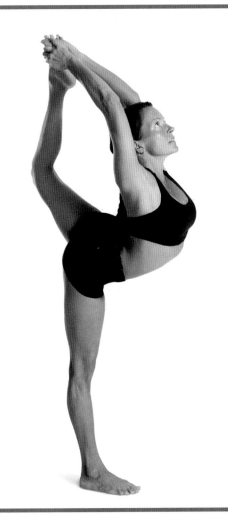

HOW TO GET THERE:

- Begin standing at the top of the mat.
- Bend your left knee, and bring your left heel toward your left gluteus.
- Externally rotate your left foot, and with your left palm facing up, reach your hand for the inside blade of your foot.
- Drop your left elbow down to find the foot bind, and rotate up to the ceiling as you kick your foot into your hand.
- Once your left elbow is pointing up, reach your arm overhead and grab your left forearm or toes.

WHERE TO ENGAGE:

- Press your hand and foot together to move into the backbend.
- Lift up through your left heel.
- Reach your elbows up and back.
- Lift through your chest.
- Squeeze your right quadriceps to straighten the standing leg.
- Ground down into all four corners of your right foot.

ANATOMY NOTES/TIPS & TRICKS:

- Keep your hips square to the mat.
- Don't pull your foot forward to deepen the backbend. Instead, reach your elbows up, and keep them in line with your shoulders. Reach through your chest to deepen the backbend.
- This is a very deep backbend. Use a strap if the pose is not accessible, and begin to practice walking your hands down the strap toward your foot as your body becomes more open.

DANCER ADVANCED ASANA:
OUTSIDE HALF BOW BOUND HALF MOON *(Chapasana)*

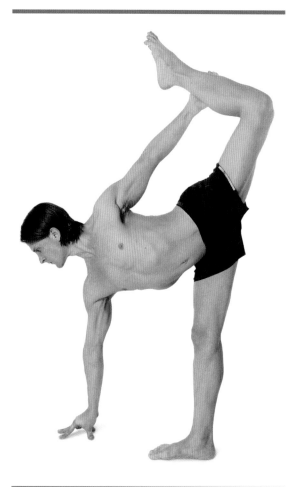

HOW TO GET THERE:

- Begin in dancer on the right side.
- Begin to lean forward and lower your right fingertips toward the mat. Keep your left hand wrapped around the inside of your left foot.
- Once your fingertips reach the mat, bring your palm down flat, and open your hips so that your left hip stacks on top of your right.
- Reach your left heel away from your butt.

WHERE TO ENGAGE:

- Press down firmly through all four corners of the standing leg.
- Fire through your left quadriceps to get deeper into the backbend.
- Rotate your chest open toward the ceiling.

ANATOMY NOTES/TIPS & TRICKS:

- The more you kick your hand and foot together, the more it will be necessary to counter this by shifting your hips in the opposite direction.
- Gaze straight ahead or toward the ceiling.
- Balance on your fingertips, or use a block under your right hand if your right hamstring is too tight to find the pose.

4

Inverted Poses

In the yoga world, the word *inversion* connotes having your head lower than your heart. An inversion can be anything from down dog to forward fold to headstand, and we've already covered many of those types of inversions in this book so far.

In this section, we build on that base as we cover the basics of how to perform crane/crow, headstand, handstand, and shoulder stand as well as advanced variations of each of these poses.

GATEWAY POSE:
CRANE/CROW

Crane/crow is often one of the first arm balances mastered. It's a fun and accessible pose that requires a mix of trust, body awareness, and strength.

Many new students believe they do not possess the upper body strength to perform crane pose, but it's less about strength and more about technique and total body engagement. In this chapter, progressions are provided for mastering crow pose as well as advanced variations such as a one-leg crow, transitioning to tripod headstand and back to crow, and jumping back through chaturanga.

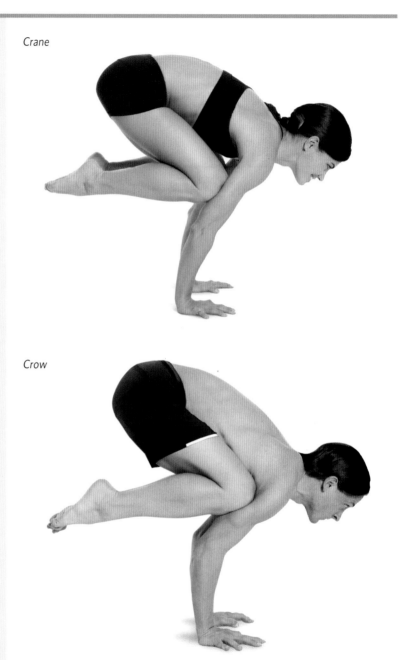

Crane

Crow

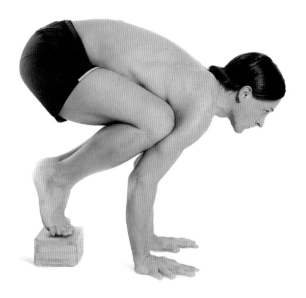

HOW TO GET THERE:

- Begin in a standing position at the top of the mat.

- Squat down and bring your palms to the floor and begin to bend your knees and your elbows.

- Stack your knees on top of your triceps as close to your armpits as possible. Bring your toes in and touch them together if possible.

- Shift weight forward into your fingertips and lift your toes off the floor and heels toward your gluteus.

- For crane pose, straighten your arms completely. For crow pose, elbows can stay bent.

WHERE TO ENGAGE:

- Bring a lot of weight forward and really press into your palms, grip into your fingertips, and lift up through your chest.

- Squeeze your elbows in like you would in a chaturanga, staying very active in your arms.

- Draw your heels toward your butt and create an active lift through your legs.

- Draw your abdominal wall in and up to help support the weight of your body in the arm balance.

ANATOMY NOTES/ TIPS & TRICKS:

- Shift more weight forward than you think is necessary and feel the weight in your palms and fingertips.

- Envision your whole body engaging and lifting up. Nothing should be loose or disengaged here.

- If you are struggling with the arm balance, place your feet on a block and your palms on the floor. This helps get you into the proper position for crow, and you can begin to practice lifting one foot off the block and then two for the arm balance.

CRANE/CROW ARM BALANCE:
ONE- LEG CROW *(Eka Pada Bakasana)*

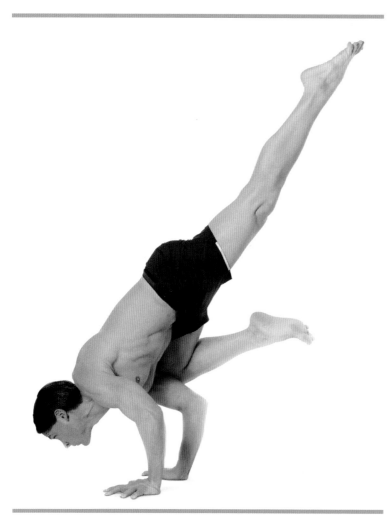

- Draw your abdominal wall in and up to help support the weight of your body in the arm balance.

- Firmly fire through your left quadriceps to straighten your leg behind you.

ANATOMY NOTES/ TIPS & TRICKS:

- This is a difficult variation of crow that requires strength and trust. Get comfortable hovering your knee off your tricep before attempting to straighten your leg behind you.

- Shift more weight forward than you think is necessary and feel the weight in your palms and fingertips.

- Envision your whole body engaging and lifting up. Nothing should be loose or disengaged here.

HOW TO GET THERE:

- Begin in crow pose.

- Shift weight to your right side and start to feel lightness in your left side.

- Lift your left knee off of your left tricep and hover.

- As you feel ready, straighten your left leg behind you.

WHERE TO ENGAGE:

- Really feel the transfer of weight to your right side, and feel solid and stable in your right side.

- Squeeze your elbows in like you would in a chaturanga, staying very active in your arms.

CRANE/CROW INVERSION:
HEADSTAND *(Salamba Shirshasana)*
AND BACK TO CROW

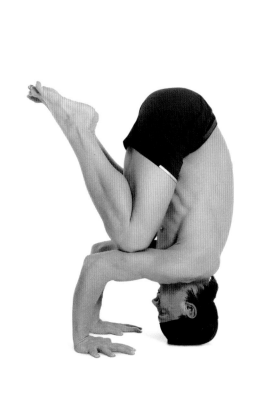 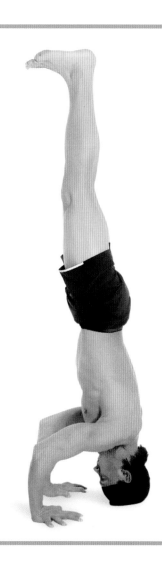

(continued on next page)

CRANE/CROW INVERSION:

HEADSTAND AND BACK TO CROW

(continued)

HOW TO GET THERE:

- Begin in crow.

- Shift even more weight forward, tuck your chin, and place the crown of your head on the floor. Squeeze your elbows in line with your shoulders, and keep your knees stacked on your triceps.

- Come into a tripod position on the floor with your palms flat on the floor and your knees resting on top of your triceps. Your hips should be stacked over your shoulders.

- Slowly lift your knees off your triceps, and come into a headstand with straight legs.

WHERE TO ENGAGE:

- Squeeze your quadriceps and inner thighs to stay active in your legs.

- Your abdominals and obliques should be kept engaged throughout.

ANATOMY NOTES/ TIPS & TRICKS:

- Form an equilateral triangle between your hands and head. This means that the distance between your hands should match the distance between either hand and your head, just like a tripod.

- Keep the weight of this pose equally distributed between your head and hands for the greatest feeling of stability.

- Your chin should be in a neutral position to ensure your neck is in alignment.

- To come out of the inversion, hinge at your waist and slowly bring your legs down toward the floor. Place your knees back on your triceps, and shift weight onto your fingertips. Lift back into crow pose.

CRANE/CROW INVERSION:
HANDSTAND PRESS

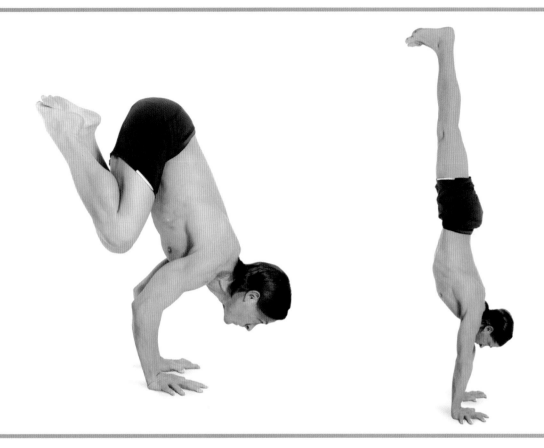

HOW TO GET THERE:

- Begin in crow.

- Shift weight forward, and stack your hips over your shoulders. Keep your knees close to your chest, and allow them to begin to lift up and leave your triceps as you move forward.

- Extend your legs straight up overhead, and bring your body into a straight line from heels to hips to shoulders to wrists.

WHERE TO ENGAGE:

- Actively flex your abdominal muscles to prevent backward momentum and your gluteus maximus to prevent yourself from folding forward at your waist and coming down.

- Engage your triceps to keep your elbows in full extension.

- Squeeze your inner thighs to keep your legs together.

ANATOMY NOTES/ TIPS & TRICKS:

- Keep your gaze between your hands or slightly in front of your fingertips throughout.

- Your shoulders will be in front of your wrists when you are in crow pose, so as you straighten your body into handstand, be sure to shift your shoulders back over your wrists.

- For a big challenge, try to move back into crow from handstand.

CROW ADVANCED ASANA:
JUMP BACK CHATURANGA

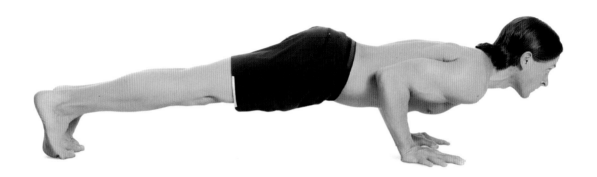

HOW TO GET THERE:

- Begin in crow pose.
- Lift your knees off your triceps, and shoot your legs straight back behind you.
- Land in a low plank position like you are in the bottom of your chaturanga with your elbows in and bent at 90 degrees.
- Move through upward facing dog to down dog to complete the vinyasa.

WHERE TO ENGAGE:

- Draw your abdominals in and up to help float your knees off your triceps.
- Fire through your quadriceps to shoot your legs back and extend them long.
- Squeeze your elbows into your side body as you come into the chaturanga position.

ANATOMY NOTES/ TIPS & TRICKS:

- This is one of those transitions where you have to trust yourself and go for it. The key is getting your knees off your triceps and sending your legs back quickly. Landing in a low plank position makes for a softer transition through chaturanga.

GATEWAY POSE:
HEADSTAND

The ability to perform a headstand often serves as a huge benchmark in a student's practice. Mastering this pose requires consistent practice, body awareness, and a willing attitude.

Start practicing headstands by getting comfortable balancing with your knees on your triceps and getting your hips over your shoulders. Once that becomes comfortable, lift your legs into headstand, but use a wall for support. Eventually build the confidence to move off the wall.

Once you can confidently perform a basic headstand, there are numerous different arm and leg placements to try. The variations shown in this chapter range from beginner to advanced.

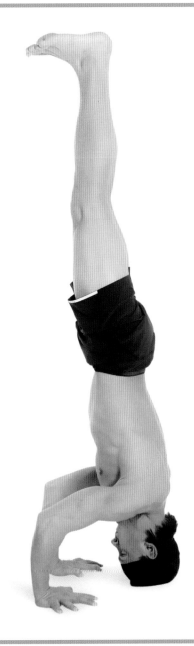

HEADSTAND ADVANCED ASANA:
TRIPOD HEADSTAND

HOW TO GET THERE:

- Begin in down dog.

- Drop to your hands and knees, and place the crown of your head on the floor as far out in front of you as your hands are apart.

- Tuck your toes and lift your hips.

- Begin to walk forward until your hips are slightly in front of your shoulders and your feet leave the ground.

- Keeping your legs glued together, lift both legs straight up overhead. Stack your hips over your shoulders, and form a straight line from head to toe.

- Keep your gaze forward on one single point.

WHERE TO ENGAGE:

- Squeeze your inner thighs together.

- Abdominals and obliques should be kept active throughout.

- Engage your gluteus maximus to prevent breaking at your waist.

ANATOMY NOTES/
TIPS & TRICKS:

- Form an equilateral triangle between your hands and head. This means that the distance between your hands should match the distance between either hand and your head, just like a tripod.

- Keep the weight of this pose equally distributed between your head and hands for the greatest sense of stability.

- Your chin should be in a neutral position to ensure your neck is in alignment.

- In order for your legs to lift off the mat, your hips must move forward in front of your shoulders to counter their weight. This requires extremely strong abdominal control and is perhaps the most difficult aspect of this pose.

- An easier alternative is to lift one leg up, drawing one knee into your chest followed by the other, and then lifting both legs simultaneously from the bent-knee position.

- Avoid kicking into this posture and relying on momentum; this could compromise the safety of your neck.

- Flex your toes toward your shins, and try to feel like you are standing on the ceiling.

- Your heels should stack over your knees, knees over hips, and hips over shoulders.

HEADSTAND ADVANCED ASANA:
PIKE *(Urdhva Dandasana A)*

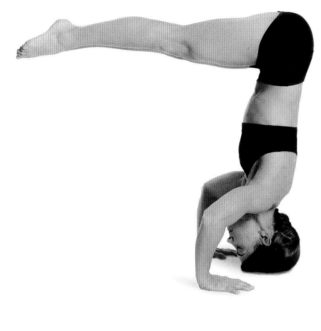

HOW TO GET THERE:

- Begin in headstand.
- Hinge at your waist, and lower your legs halfway down into a pike position. Your body will be in an L-shape.

WHERE TO ENGAGE:

- Squeeze your inner thighs together.
- Your abdominals and obliques should be kept active throughout.

ANATOMY NOTES/ TIPS & TRICKS:

- Keep the weight of this pose equally distributed between your head and hands for the greatest sense of stability.
- Your chin should be in a neutral position to ensure your neck is in alignment.
- Keep your elbows squeezing in and aligned with your shoulders.

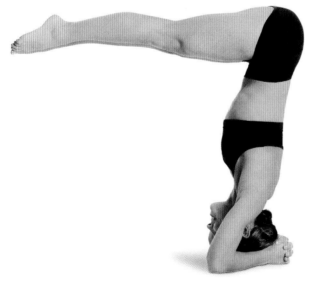

HEADSTAND ADVANCED ASANA:
REVOLVED HIPS *(Parsva-Sirsasana)*

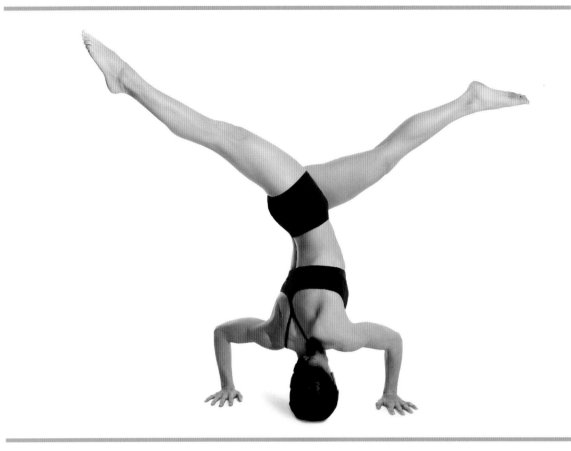

HOW TO GET THERE:

- Begin in headstand.

- Maintain the same alignment from your waist down to your shoulders.

- From your waist down to your feet, begin to rotate so that your feet face the right side of your mat. Pause for a few breaths.

- Repeat, rotating so that your feet face the left side of your mat. Again, pause for a few breaths.

WHERE TO ENGAGE:

- Your abdominals and obliques should be kept active throughout.

- Engage your gluteus maximus to prevent breaking at your waist.

- Squeeze your quadriceps to keep your legs straight.

ANATOMY NOTES/ TIPS & TRICKS:

- Keep your upper body and core engaged and in your normal handstand position. Your hips and legs should be the only things moving here.

- Don't rely on momentum. Move intentionally and slowly.

HEADSTAND ADVANCED ASANA:
SPLIT LEGS *(Parivrittaikapada Shirshasana)*

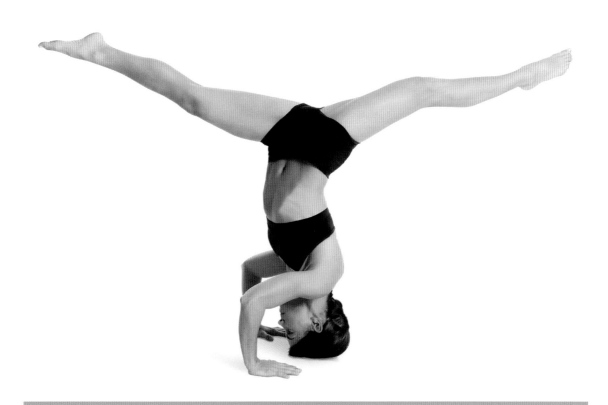

HOW TO GET THERE:

- Begin in headstand.
- Maintain the same alignment from your waist down to your shoulders.
- With straight legs, reach your right leg toward the top of the mat, while your left leg reaches toward the back of the mat until both legs are parallel to the mat.

WHERE TO ENGAGE:

- Squeeze your inner thighs, spiraling internally.
- Your abdominals and obliques should be kept active throughout.

ANATOMY NOTES/ TIPS & TRICKS:

- With your legs spread in this position, many practitioners find that it is much easier to balance.

HEADSTAND ADVANCED ASANA:
LOTUS PREP *(Padma Shirshasana)*

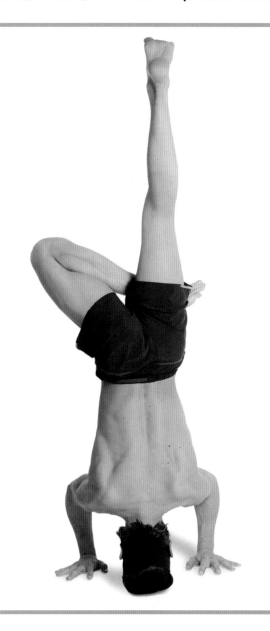

HOW TO GET THERE:

- Begin in headstand.
- Begin to bend your right knee, bringing your right foot toward the top of your left thigh.
- Crawl your right foot into the crease of your left thigh until it is securely into a lotus position.
- Point your right knee upward and your left leg straight.

WHERE TO ENGAGE:

- Draw the right heel of your foot downward and toward your navel.
- Your abdominals and obliques should be kept active throughout.
- Engage your left gluteus maximus to prevent breaking at your waist.

ANATOMY NOTES/TIPS & TRICKS:

- While you draw your right heel into lotus, it can make it easier if you bend at your waist, allow your hips to move slightly in front of your shoulders, and draw your left knee downward to help push your right foot into place.

HEADSTAND ADVANCED ASANA:
FULL LOTUS *(Padma Shirshasana)*

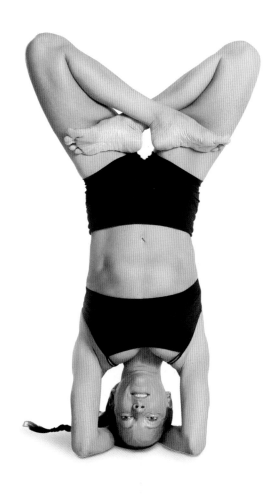

HOW TO GET THERE:

- Begin in headstand.

- Begin to bend your right knee, bringing your right foot toward the top of your left thigh.

- Bend at your waist, allow your hips to move slightly in front of your shoulders, and draw your left knee downward to help push your right foot into place, while crawling your right foot into the crease of your left thigh until it is securely in a lotus position.

- Bend your left knee, and draw your left foot onto your upper right thigh and upward until it is securely in the lotus position.

WHERE TO ENGAGE:

- Draw the heels of your feet downward and toward your navel.

- Your abdominals and obliques should be kept active throughout.

- Engage your gluteus maximus to prevent breaking at your waist.

- Squeeze your knees in toward one another using your inner thighs.

ANATOMY NOTES/TIPS & TRICKS:

- Try not to rely on strength when transitioning into lotus, but rather soften into it. Remain at ease while positioning your feet on top of your thighs. Once a foot is on top of a thigh, you will have more leverage and can be a little more engaged in your legs.

HEADSTAND ADVANCED ASANA:
ARMS-EXTENDED HEADSTAND
(Mukta Hasta Sirsasana B)

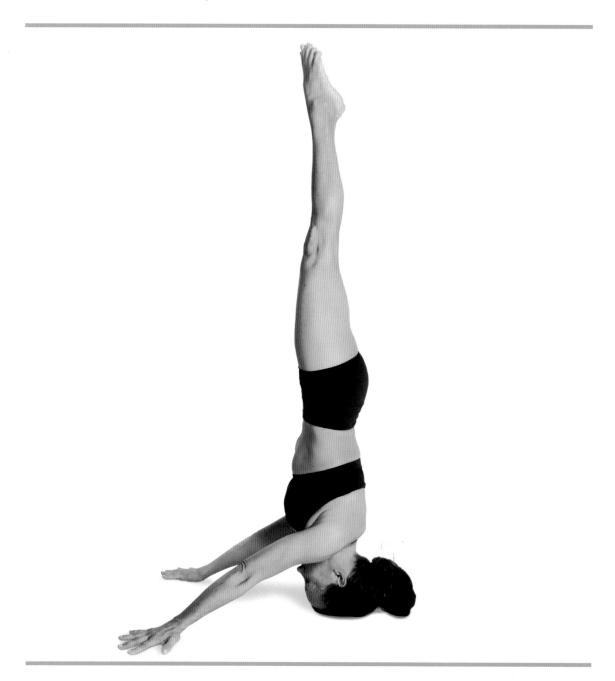

HOW TO GET THERE:

- Begin in down dog.

- Drop to your knees, tuck your chin, place the crown of your head on the floor about a foot in front of your knees, and extend both arms out in front of you and off slightly to an angle outside shoulder width. The backs of your hands should press down with your palms facing upward.

- Tuck your toes and lift your hips.

- Press firmly into the backs of your hands, and keep your arms straight.

- Begin to walk forward until your hips are slightly in front of your shoulders and your feet leave the ground.

- Lift your legs parallel to the floor into a "pike" position.

- Once you're stable, begin lifting your legs straight up as your hips realign directly over your shoulders.

- Keep your gaze forward on one single point.

WHERE TO ENGAGE:

- Squeeze your inner thighs together.

- Your abdominals and obliques should be kept active throughout.

- Engage your gluteus maximus to prevent breaking at your waist.

ANATOMY NOTES/ TIPS & TRICKS:

- A significant amount of load-bearing weight will be on your neck. Make sure to keep your chin in a neutral position to ensure your neck is in alignment.

- In order for your legs to lift off the mat, your hips must move forward in front of your shoulders to counter their weight. This requires extremely strong abdominal control and is perhaps the most difficult aspect of this pose.

- An easier alternative is to lift one leg up first, drawing one knee into your chest followed by the other, and then lifting both legs simultaneously from the bent-knee position.

- Avoid kicking into this posture and relying on momentum because this could compromise the safety of your neck.

- Flex your toes toward your shins, and try to feel like you are standing on the ceiling.

- Your heels should stack over your knees, knees over hips, and hips over shoulders.

HEADSTAND ADVANCED ASANA:
WIDE ARMS—EXTENDED HEADSTAND
(Mukta Hasta Sirsasana C)

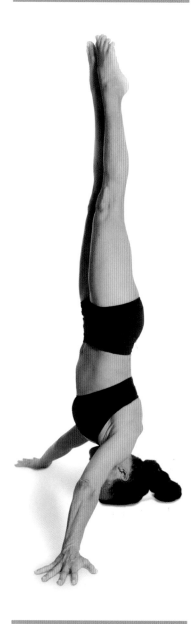

HOW TO GET THERE:

- Begin in down dog.

- Drop to your knees, tuck your chin, place the crown of your head on the floor about a foot in front of your knees, and extend both arms out to the side of you, angled slightly so that your hands are still visible in your peripheral vision.

- Tuck your toes and lift your hips.

- Press firmly into your hands, and keep your arms straight.

- Begin to walk forward until your hips are slightly in front of your shoulders and your feet leave the ground.

- Lift your legs parallel to the floor into a "pike" position.

- Once you're stable, begin lifting your legs straight up as your hips realign directly over your shoulders.

- Keep your gaze forward on one single point.

WHERE TO ENGAGE:

- Squeeze your inner thighs together.

- Your abdominals and obliques should be kept active throughout.

- Engage your gluteus maximus to prevent breaking at your waist.

ANATOMY NOTES/ TIPS & TRICKS:

- A significant amount of load-bearing weight will be on your neck. Make sure to keep your chin in a neutral position to ensure your neck is in alignment.

- In order for your legs to lift off the mat, your hips must move forward in front of your shoulders to counter their weight. This requires extremely strong abdominal control and is perhaps the most difficult aspect of this pose.

- An easier alternative is to lift one leg up first, drawing one knee into your chest followed by the other, and then lifting both legs simultaneously from the bent-knee position.

- Avoid kicking into this posture and relying on momentum. This could compromise the safety of your neck.

- Flex your toes toward your shins, and try to feel like you are standing on the ceiling.

- Your heels should stack over your knees, knees over hips, and hips over shoulders.

- Keep the weight of this pose equally distributed between your head and hands for the greatest sense of stability.

HEADSTAND ADVANCED ASANA:
BOUND FOREARM BALANCING HEADSTAND
(Baddha Hasta Sirsasana A)

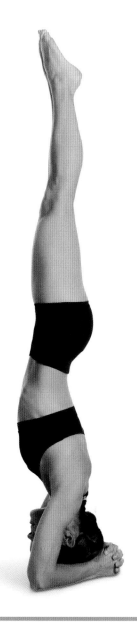

HOW TO GET THERE:

- Begin in down dog.

- Drop to your hands and knees, and come down onto your forearms.

- Interlace your fingers and press your palms firmly together.

- Tuck your chin, and place the crown of your head in between your forearms so that the back of your head rests against your hands.

- Tuck your toes and lift your hips.

- Begin to walk forward until your hips are slightly in front of your shoulders and your feet leave the ground.

- Lift your legs parallel to the floor into a "pike" position.

- Keep your gaze forward on one single point.

- Once you're stable, begin lifting your legs straight up as your hips realign directly over your shoulders.

WHERE TO ENGAGE:

- Keep your palms sealed tightly.

- Press firmly into your forearms.

- Squeeze your inner thighs together.

- Your abdominals and obliques should be kept active throughout.

- Engage your gluteus maximus to prevent breaking at your waist.

ANATOMY NOTES/ TIPS & TRICKS:

- A significant amount of load-bearing weight will be on your neck. Make sure to keep your chin in a neutral position to ensure your neck is in alignment.

- In order for your legs to lift off the mat, your hips must move forward in front of your shoulders to counter their weight. This requires extremely strong abdominal control and is perhaps the most difficult aspect of this pose.

- An easier alternative is to lift one leg up first, drawing one knee into your chest followed by the other, and then lifting both legs simultaneously from the bent-knee position.

- Avoid kicking into this posture and relying on momentum. This could compromise the safety of your neck.

- Flex your toes toward your shins, and try to feel like you are standing on the ceiling.

- Your heels should stack over your knees, knees over hips, and hips over shoulders.

HEADSTAND ADVANCED ASANA:
CROSSED ARMS HEADSTAND
(Baddha Hasta Sirsasana B)

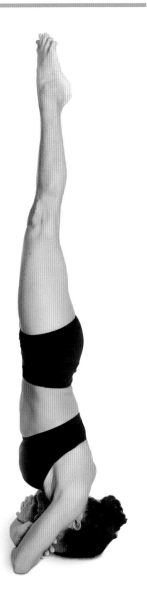

HOW TO GET THERE:

- Begin in down dog.

- Drop to your hands and knees, and come down onto your forearms.

- Cross your arms so your right hand and forearm are stacked and sealed in front of your left hand and forearm.

- Tuck your chin, and place the crown of your head as far out in front of your arms as it will reach, without your arms leaving their position.

- Tuck your toes and lift your hips.

- Balancing on the crown of your head and your forearms, begin to walk forward until your hips are slightly in front of your shoulders and your feet leave the ground.

- Lift your legs parallel to the floor into a "pike" position.

- Keep your gaze forward on one single point.

- Once you're stable, begin lifting your legs straight up as your hips realign directly over your shoulders.

WHERE TO ENGAGE:

- Keep your palms sealed tightly.

- Press firmly into your forearms.

- Squeeze your inner thighs together.

- Your abdominals and obliques should be kept active throughout.

- Engage your gluteus maximus to prevent breaking at your waist.

ANATOMY NOTES/ TIPS & TRICKS:

- A significant amount of load-bearing weight will be on your neck. Make sure to keep your chin in a neutral position to ensure your neck is in alignment.

- In order for your legs to lift off the mat, your hips must move forward in front of your shoulders to counter their weight. This requires extremely strong abdominal control and is perhaps the most difficult aspect of this pose.

- An easier alternative is to lift one leg up first, drawing one knee into your chest followed by the other, and then lifting both legs simultaneously from the bent-knee position.

- Avoid kicking into this posture and relying on momentum. This could compromise the safety of your neck.

- Flex your toes toward your shins, and try to feel like you are standing on the ceiling.

- Your heels should stack over your knees, knees over hips, and hips over shoulders.

HEADSTAND ADVANCED ASANA:
FOREARM BALANCING HEADSTAND
(Baddha Hasta Sirsasana C)

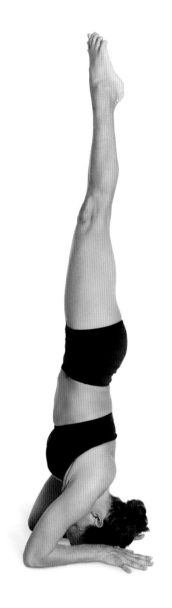

HOW TO GET THERE:

- Begin in down dog.

- Drop to your hands and knees, and come down onto your forearms.

- Keep your palms flat and forearms parallel while you tuck your chin and place the crown of your head in between your hands. Your forearms remain on the ground.

- Tuck your toes and lift your hips.

- Balancing on the crown of your head and your forearms, begin to walk forward until your hips are slightly in front of your shoulders and your feet leave the ground.

- Lift your legs parallel to the floor into a "pike" position.

- Keep your gaze forward on one single point.

- Once you're stable, begin lifting your legs straight up as your hips realign directly over your shoulders.

WHERE TO ENGAGE:

- Keep your palms sealed tightly.

- Press firmly into your forearms.

- Squeeze your inner thighs together.

- Your abdominals and obliques should be kept active throughout.

- Engage your gluteus maximus to prevent breaking at your waist.

ANATOMY NOTES/ TIPS & TRICKS:

- A significant amount of load-bearing weight will be on your neck. Make sure to keep your chin in a neutral position to ensure your neck is in alignment.

- In order for your legs to lift off the mat, your hips must move forward in front of your shoulders to counter their weight. This requires extremely strong abdominal control and is perhaps the most difficult aspect of this pose.

- An easier alternative is to lift one leg up first, drawing one knee into your chest followed by the other, and then lifting both legs simultaneously from the bent-knee position.

- Avoid kicking into this posture and relying on momentum. This could compromise the safety of your neck.

- Flex your toes toward your shins, and try to feel like you are standing on the ceiling.

- Your heels should stack over your knees, knees over hips, and hips over shoulders.

HEADSTAND ADVANCED ASANA:
PALMS TO SHOULDER HEADSTAND
(Baddha Hasta Sirsasana D)

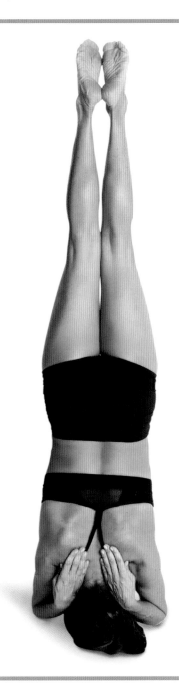

HOW TO GET THERE:

- Begin in down dog.

- Drop to your hands and knees, and come down onto your forearms.

- Keep your palms flat and your forearms parallel while you tuck your chin and place the crown of your head in between your forearms so that your hands are slightly in front of your head.

- Turn your palms face up and place them underneath your shoulders.

- Tuck your toes and lift your hips.

- Balancing on the crown of your head and your elbows, begin to walk forward until your hips are slightly in front of your shoulders and your feet leave the ground.

- Lift your legs parallel to the floor into a "pike" position.

- Keep your gaze forward on one single point.

- Once you're stable, begin lifting your legs straight up as your hips realign directly over your shoulders.

WHERE TO ENGAGE:

- Keep your palms sealed tightly.

- Press firmly into your forearms.

- Squeeze your inner thighs together.

- Your abdominals and obliques should be kept active throughout.

- Engage your gluteus maximus to prevent breaking at your waist.

ANATOMY NOTES/ TIPS & TRICKS:

- A significant amount of load-bearing weight will be on your neck. Make sure to keep your chin in a neutral position to ensure your neck is in alignment.

- In order for your legs to lift off the mat, your hips must move forward in front of your shoulders to counter their weight. This requires extremely strong abdominal control and is perhaps the most difficult aspect of this pose.

- An easier alternative is to lift one leg up first, drawing one knee into your chest followed by the other, and then lifting both legs simultaneously from the bent-knee position.

- Avoid kicking into this posture and relying on momentum. This could compromise the safety of your neck.

- Flex your toes toward your shins, and try to feel like you are standing on the ceiling.

- Your heels should stack over your knees, knees over hips, and hips over shoulders.

HANDSTAND *(Adho Mukha Vrksasana)*

Handstands are the ultimate inversion thanks to the combination of strength, body awareness, self-confidence, and grace that they provide. Many students consider them out of reach, but with time, practice, and dedication, they are accessible.

These are basic instructions for getting into a handstand pose and variations of it. There are alternate gateways into it covered in this book, including jumping from down dog, pressing from forward fold, lifting from standing splits, pressing from wide leg forward fold, and pressing from crow.

Get playful with your handstands, and remember—practice makes progress! If you want handstands, you must practice them regularly!

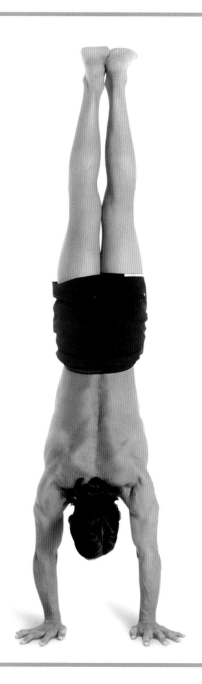

HOW TO GET THERE:

- Begin in a forward fold, and lift your left leg to standing split.

- With both palms flat on the floor, gaze forward in front of your right foot, and lift your chest slightly off your thigh to lengthen your spine.

- Shift weight onto the ball of your right foot, and begin to take some small hops, lifting your left leg toward the ceiling and allowing your right toes to leave the mat.

- Once you find a balance point where your hips stack over your shoulders, bring your right leg up to meet your left.

WHERE TO ENGAGE:

- The lift and engagement of your left leg is crucial for getting into handstand position.

- Actively flex your abdominal muscles to prevent backward momentum and your gluteus maximus to prevent yourself from folding forward at your waist and coming down.

- Engage your triceps to keep your elbows in full extension.

- Squeeze your inner thighs to keep your legs together.

ANATOMY NOTES/ TIPS & TRICKS:

- Keep your gaze between your hands or past your fingertips.

- The goal is to form a straight line from your hands to your feet, so the engagement of your abdominals and your gluteus maximus is imperative. It's common to have a sway in your lower back, so really press out of your shoulders, squeeze your abdominals, and drop your tailbone to prevent that.

- The tendency here is to want to use force to kick up into handstand. Use body awareness and control instead. The key to lifting into the handstand is getting your hips stacked over your shoulders. Practice taking small hops and really lifting through your left leg to get into this position. Once your hips are over your shoulders, lifting up to handstand is simple.

- Perform your handstands against a wall for support until you can confidently lift into the inversion and feel comfortable holding the position on your own. On a related note, don't become dependent on the wall, and trust yourself to try handstands away from it once you've mastered the pose on the wall.

HANDSTAND ADVANCED ASANA:
HANDSTAND SPLITS *(Adho Mukha Vrksasana)*

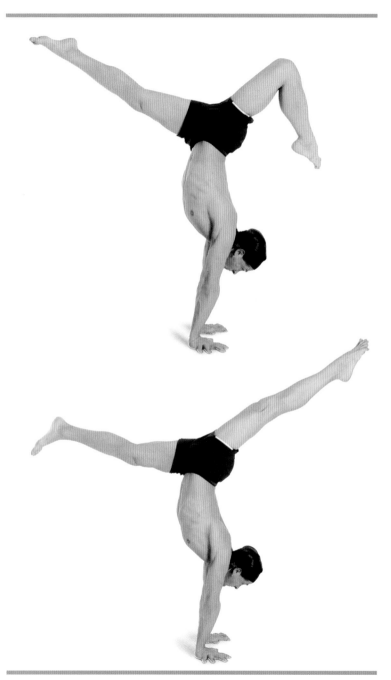

HOW TO GET THERE:

- Begin in handstand.

- Maintain the same alignment from your waist down to your shoulders.

- With your legs straight, reach your right leg toward the top of the mat, while your left leg reaches toward the back of the mat until both legs are parallel to the mat.

WHERE TO ENGAGE:

- Squeeze your inner thighs, spiraling internally.

- Your abdominals and obliques should be kept active throughout.

ANATOMY NOTES/
TIPS & TRICKS:

- With your legs spread in this position, many practitioners find that it is much easier to balance.

- Bend one or both knees for a fun and visually interesting variation of the pose.

HANDSTAND ADVANCED ASANA:
HANDSTAND SCORPION *(Vrischikasana II)*

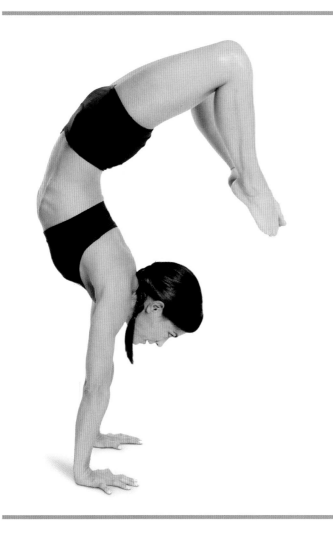

HOW TO GET THERE:

- Begin in handstand.

- Gaze forward, looking straight out in front of you.

- Pull your chest through your shoulders as you bend both knees, and reach the tips of your toes toward the back of your head.

WHERE TO ENGAGE:

- Spread your fingers wide and press down through your fingertips.

- Squeeze your hamstrings to get your toes closer to the back of your head.

ANATOMY NOTES/ TIPS & TRICKS:

- When you lift your gaze forward, be mindful to keep your neck long.

- Actively think about pulling your heart center forward and tucking your pelvis under.

GATEWAY POSE:

SHOULDER STAND *(Salamba Sarvangasana)*

Shoulder stand is commonly included in yoga practices as one of the final postures before moving into svanasana. Shoulder stand has long been regarded as an extremely therapeutic inversion. Its benefits include strengthening the upper body, conditioning the core and lower body, helping with insomnia, reducing stress and anxiety, improved digestion, and more.

Full shoulder stand can be difficult for some, so if you feel any strain in the neck or spine or general discomfort in the posture, try the half shoulder stand variation included in this chapter before moving on to the more intense variations.

The key to all shoulder stands is making sure that the weight of the body is resting on the shoulders, as the pose name implies, and not on the neck and spine.

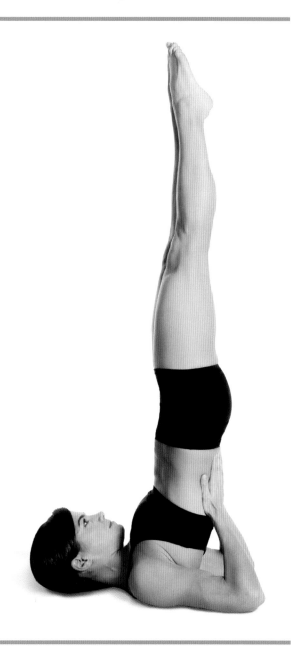

HOW TO GET THERE:

- Start by lying flat on your back with your legs extended and your arms by your sides.

- Lift both legs perpendicular to the floor.

- Press both palms flat into the floor, and lift your legs upward so that your hips come off the floor.

- With your hips lifted, place your palms at the small of your lower back, bend your elbows and squeeze them toward one another, and support the weight of your hips and legs in an inverted position.

- Begin to draw your hips over your shoulders, and reach upward through your heels, forming a vertical line.

WHERE TO ENGAGE:

- Abdominals must engage to lift your hips off the floor and upward.

- Your scapulae retract as you squeeze your elbows together and allow your shoulders to externally rotate; this is made possible through engaging your middle trapezius and rhomboids.

ANATOMY NOTES/ TIPS & TRICKS:

- This pose places your cervical spine into a flexed position. While the final expression of this pose is to have a vertical line from your feet to your shoulders, for beginners being introduced to this pose, there are still benefits from spending time in it with a slight bend at your waist so that your neck bears less weight.

- In order to get your shoulders fully retracted, it may be helpful to interlace your hands together into a bind. Once bound, you can press down into your hands for support while you walk your shoulders closer together.

- Another variation is to start in halasana (plow pose) with your hands already bound, and to lift your legs vertically from there.

SHOULDER STAND ADVANCED ASANA:
HALF SHOULDER STAND *(Ardha Sarvangasana)*

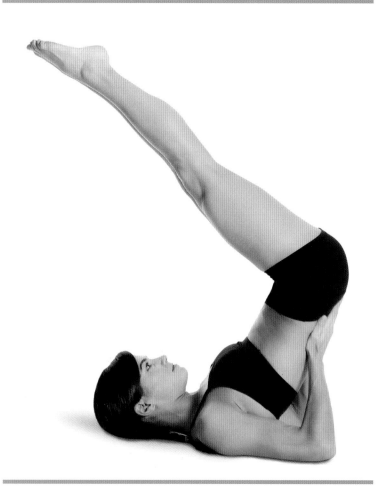

WHERE TO ENGAGE:

- Your abdominals must engage to lift your hips off the floor and upward.

- Your scapulae retract as you squeeze your elbows together and allow your shoulders to externally rotate; this is made possible through engaging your middle trapezius and rhomboids.

ANATOMY NOTES/ TIPS & TRICKS:

- This can be a very restorative and relaxing posture with the support of blocks or blankets. Rather than using your arms for support under your lower back, place blocks or blankets underneath you to the desired elevation, while your legs remain over your hips and your arms are by your sides.

HOW TO GET THERE:

- Start by lying flat on your back with your legs extended and your arms by your sides.

- Lift both legs perpendicular to the floor.

- Press both palms flat into the floor, and lift your legs upward so that your hips come off the floor.

- With your hips lifted, place your palms at the small of your lower back, bend your elbows and squeeze them toward one another, and support the weight of your hips and legs in an inverted position.

SHOULDER STAND ADVANCED ASANA:
ONE LEG SUPPORTED SHOULDER STAND
(Eka Pada Sarvangasana)

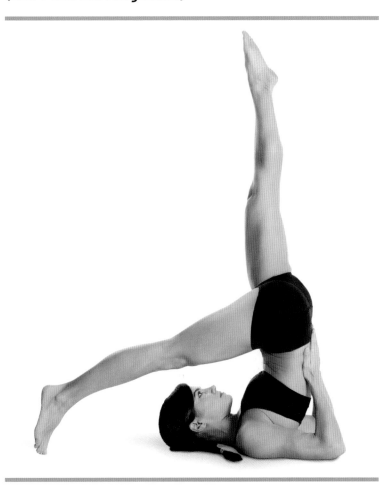

ANATOMY NOTES/ TIPS & TRICKS:

- This pose places your cervical spine into a flexed position. While the final expression of this pose is to have a vertical line from your feet to your shoulders, for beginners being introduced to this pose, there are still benefits from spending time in it with a slight bend at your waist so that your neck bears less weight.

- In order to get your shoulders fully retracted, it may be helpful to interlace your hands together into a bind. Once bound, you can press down into your hands for support while you walk your shoulders closer together.

- It can be helpful, if your hamstrings are tight, to flex the foot of the one that is lowered to the floor toward your shin.

- Another variation is to start in halasana (plow pose) with your hands already bound and to lift your leg vertically from there.

HOW TO GET THERE:

- Start in shoulder stand.

- Keep your left leg vertical and, with a straight leg, lower your right overhead toward the floor with your foot pointing and your hips still stacked over your shoulders.

WHERE TO ENGAGE:

- Your abdominals must engage to lift your hips off the floor and upward.

- Your scapulae retract as you squeeze your elbows together and allow your shoulders to externally rotate; this is made possible through engaging your middle trapezius and rhomboids.

SHOULDER STAND ADVANCED ASANA:
PLOW POSE *(Halasana)*

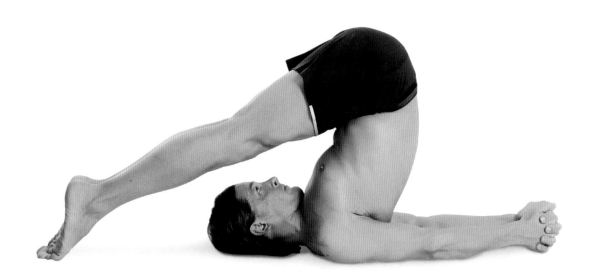

HOW TO GET THERE:

- Start in shoulder stand.

- Interlace your hands together into a bind.

- Press down into your hands for support while you walk your shoulders closer together.

- With your legs straight, lower them overhead toward the floor with your feet pointing and your hips still stacked over your shoulders.

WHERE TO ENGAGE:

- Your scapulae retract as you squeeze your elbows together and allow your shoulders to externally rotate; this is made possible through engaging your middle trapezius and rhomboids.

ANATOMY NOTES/ TIPS & TRICKS:

- It can be helpful, if your hamstrings are tight, to flex the foot of the one that is lowered to the floor toward your shin.

- Another variation is to start with your legs already overhead and to then bind your hands together before walking your shoulders together.

SHOULDER STAND ADVANCED ASANA:
DEAF MAN'S POSE *(Karnapidasana)*

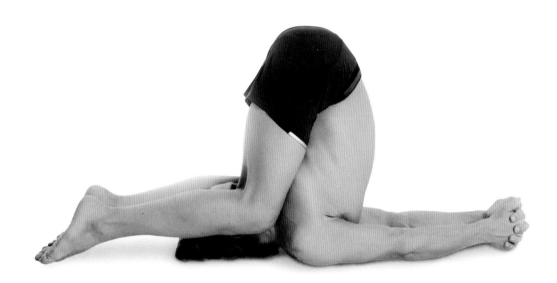

HOW TO GET THERE:

- Start in plow pose.

- Begin to bend your knees toward the floor until they are beside your ears and your shins rest on the floor.

- Squeeze your knees in toward your ears.

WHERE TO ENGAGE:

- Your abdominals must turn a lot here to fully release through your lower back in order to lower your knees toward the floor.

- Your inner thighs engage to squeeze your knees in.

ANATOMY NOTES/ TIPS & TRICKS:

- Lowering your knees and shins all the way down to the floor can take many years of practice. Lower as low as you can, and give your body time.

SHOULDER STAND ADVANCED ASANA:
LOTUS SHOULDER STAND *(Urdhva Padmasana)*

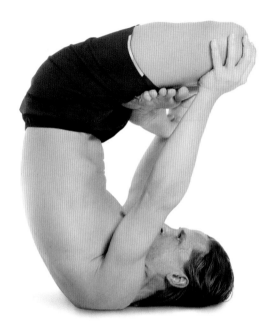

HOW TO GET THERE:

- Start in shoulder stand.

- Begin to bend your right knee, bringing your right foot toward the top of your left thigh.

- Bend at your waist, allow your hips to move slightly in front of your shoulders, and draw your left knee downward to help push your right foot into place while crawling your right foot into the crease of your left thigh until it is securely in a lotus position.

- Bend your left knee, and draw your left foot onto your upper right thigh and upward until it is securely in the lotus position.

- Place your hands on your knees, and straighten your arms as you balance on your shoulders.

WHERE TO ENGAGE:

- Squeeze through your abdominals for stability.

- Gently press your palms into your knees.

ANATOMY NOTES/ TIPS & TRICKS:

- Your lotus legs should be in a shelf-like position and parallel to the floor.

- Get comfortable holding lotus in shoulder stand before you attempt to balance with your hands at your knees.

- Tuck your chin toward your chest to lengthen your neck. Be sure to walk your shoulder blades together so that the weight is on your shoulders and not your spine.

SHOULDER STAND ADVANCED ASANA:

LOTUS SHOULDER STAND WITH BIND
(Pindasana)

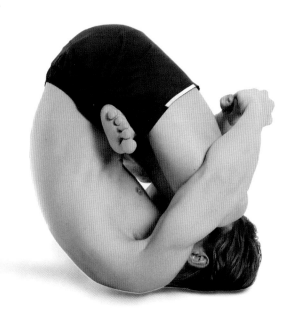

HOW TO GET THERE:

- Begin in lotus shoulder stand.

- Release your hands from your knees, and hinge at your waist to bring your knees down toward your ears.

- Wrap your arms around your legs and clasp your hands together to create a bind.

- Balance on your shoulders in the bound lotus position.

WHERE TO ENGAGE:

- Squeeze your arms into your legs to secure the bind.

ANATOMY NOTES/ TIPS & TRICKS:

- Tuck your chin toward your chest slightly to lengthen your neck.

- This can be an intense posture with the combination of the lotus legs and the bind. Soften your neck and shoulders as much as possible, and breathe into the posture.

SHOULDER STAND ADVANCED ASANA:
INVERTED WIDE LEG FOLD *(Supta Konasana)*

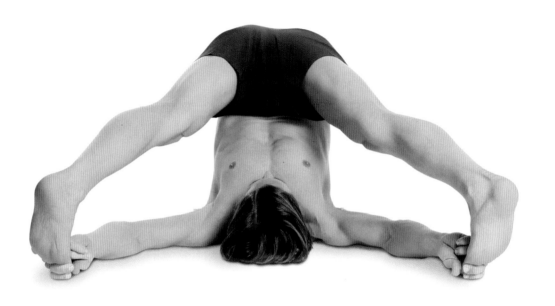

HOW TO GET THERE:

- Begin in shoulder stand.

- Keep your hands at your lower back, and hinge at your waist.

- Spread your legs wide and let your toes touch the floor behind you.

- Wrap your index and middle fingers around your big toes.

WHERE TO ENGAGE:

- Squeeze through your quadriceps to straighten your legs.

ANATOMY NOTES/ TIPS & TRICKS:

- If you need more support, keep your hands at your lower back instead of wrapping them around your toes.

- Tuck your chin slightly toward your chest to lengthen your neck.

5

Seated Poses

The fun and playfulness doesn't have to end as you reach the end of your practice. As you make your way to the floor for seated postures, there are still many variations available. In this section, we explore how to take poses such as pigeon and lotus into deeper expressions and arm balancing.

GATEWAY POSE:
SEATED PIGEON

Seated pigeon is a hip-opening pose that is widely accessible, even to those with tight hips. It serves as a nice gateway into poses such as elephant trunk, sundial, and scissors.

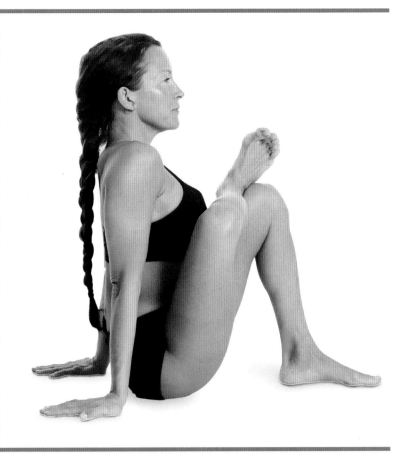

HOW TO GET THERE:

- Begin in a seated position on the mat.
- Place both palms on the floor behind you, and place your left foot flat on the floor.
- Cross your right ankle over your left knee, and sit up tall.

WHERE TO ENGAGE:

- Lift through your chest.
- Press your right knee away from you to deepen the stretch in your right hip.
- Press into your palms, and walk your hands closer to your hips to deepen the stretch. Straighten your arms if possible.

ANATOMY NOTES/ TIPS & TRICKS:

- This is a hip opener. The more you engage by sitting up tall into the posture and pressing your knee away, the deeper you will feel the stretch.
- Try to bring the right side of your gluteus down toward the mat. It will want to lift up.

SEATED PIGEON ARM BALANCE:
ELEPHANT TRUNK POSE *(Eka Hasta Bhujasana)*

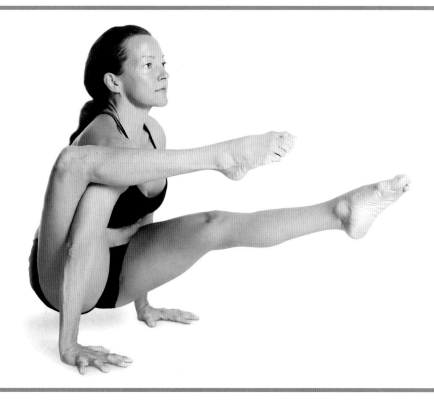

HOW TO GET THERE:

- Begin in seated pigeon on the right side.

- Drop your left knee down to the ground.

- Lean forward and bring your right thigh over your right upper tricep, and place both palms flat on the mat in line with your shoulders.

- Press into your palms to straighten your arms, and lift your hips off the floor.

- Extend your left leg straight out in front of you.

WHERE TO ENGAGE:

- Press into your palms.

- Lift up through your abdominals and your pelvic floor.

- Squeeze your left quadriceps to straighten your left leg.

ANATOMY NOTES/
TIPS & TRICKS:

- Leaning forward assists with getting your right leg over your shoulder and coming into the arm balance.

- Be sure your palms are lined up directly under your shoulders to help support the weight of your body as you balance.

SEATED PIGEON ADVANCED ASANA:
SUNDIAL *(Surya Yantrasana)*

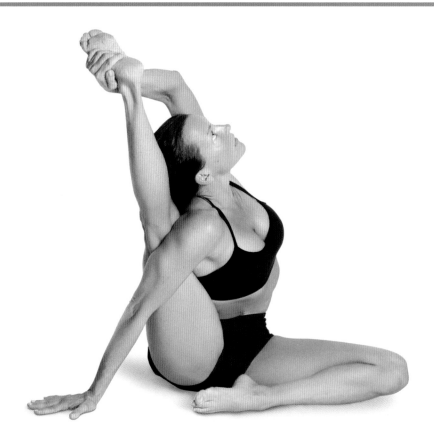

HOW TO GET THERE:

- Begin in elephant trunk pose on the right side; prep without lifting into the arm balance.

- Place your right palm flat on the mat under your right shoulder. Grab the outside blade of your right foot with your left hand.

- Reach through your right heel, and straighten your right leg as you look under your right arm.

WHERE TO ENGAGE:

- Reach through your right heel to straighten your right leg.

- Press into your right palm, and lift through your chest to sit up tall.

ANATOMY NOTES/ TIPS & TRICKS:

- Tight hamstrings can prevent you from fully straightening your right leg. Keeping your knee slightly bent will still allow you to experience the posture.

- Focus less on squeezing your quadriceps to straighten your right leg and more on reaching your heel away from you.

SEATED PIGEON ARM BALANCE:
SCISSORS *(Astavakrasana)*

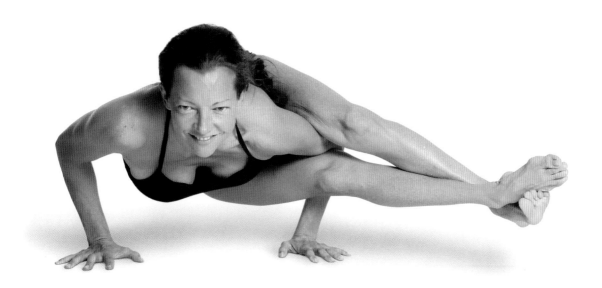

HOW TO GET THERE:

- Begin in elephant trunk pose on the right side.

- Cross your left ankle over your right, and extend your legs out to the right side.

- Lean forward and bend your arms at 90 degrees, as in chaturanga, with your hips and legs lifted off the mat.

WHERE TO ENGAGE:

- Press the floor away with your fingertips, and squeeze your elbows in.

- Engage the abdominal wall, drawing in and up.

- Once you come into scissors, squeeze your inner thighs into your arms and reach through your heels.

- Reach through your chest.

ANATOMY NOTES/ TIPS & TRICKS:

- Keep your chest and hips parallel to the floor. Squeezing your inner thighs together will facilitate this.

- Scissors is not a posture about strength. Keeping your shoulders stacked over your wrists will provide all the support you need in your arms. The strong engagement of your legs is the most vital part.

GATEWAY POSE:
PIGEON

Pigeon pose is a crowd favorite among yoga students. It addresses the tightening of the hips associated with our sitting culture and participating in sports such as running and weightlifting. Pigeon also provides emotional benefits and can help relieve stress and anxiety.

Performing a long hold in pigeon may be difficult at first. This is a pose requiring surrender and attention to breath. Once you are able to relax in the pose, try experimenting with the variations listed here.

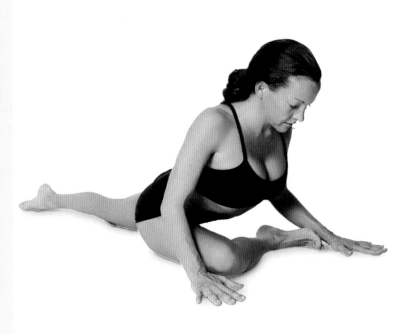

HOW TO GET THERE:

- Begin in down dog.
- Lunge your right foot to the top of the mat. Bend your knee and bring your shin across the top of the mat so that your right heel is facing the left side of the mat.
- Extend your left leg straight behind you.
- Square your hips to rest your left quadriceps on the floor.
- Begin to lean forward toward the ground, first resting on your palms, then your forearms, and finally your chest down to the floor as your body allows.

WHERE TO ENGAGE:

- Reach through your right heel, and pull your toes back toward your shin.

ANATOMY NOTES/ TIPS & TRICKS:

- Pigeon is a great hip opener that allows you to relax in the pose without having to do a lot of work.
- You eventually want to bring your right shin parallel to the top of the mat, but don't worry if you're not able to get there. Square hips are the priority here. Don't sacrifice your hip alignment to get your shin across the top of the mat.
- Make sure you're not resting on your right knee. You should be able to see it on the right side of your body when you fold forward.

PIGEON ADVANCED ASANA:
MERMAID

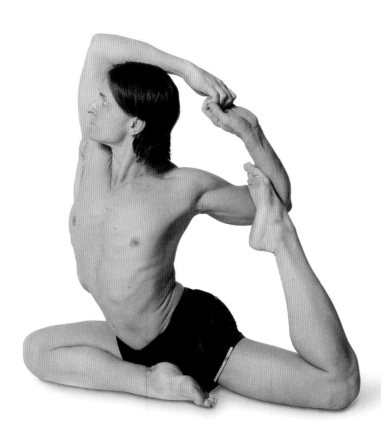

HOW TO GET THERE:

- Begin in pigeon on the left side.
- Come up to rest on your palms.
- Bend your left knee behind you, and hook your left toes into the crease of your left elbow.
- Reach your right hand overhead, and clasp your fingertips together. Point your right elbow toward the ceiling.
- Keep your hips square.

WHERE TO ENGAGE:

- Ground down through the right side of your body and your pelvis to keep your hips square.
- Lift up through your chest.

ANATOMY NOTES/ TIPS & TRICKS:

- The tendency is for the pose to collapse to the left side. Bring weight to your right side, and keep your hips square.

PIGEON ADVANCED ASANA:
KING PIGEON *(Eka Pada Rajakapotasana)*

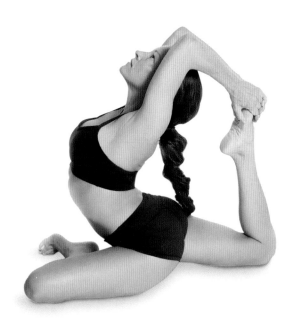

HOW TO GET THERE:

- Begin in pigeon on the right side.
- Come up to rest on your palms.
- Bend your left knee behind you, clasp your left toes with your left hand, and lift your left elbow up toward the ceiling.
- Reach your right hand back for your left toes, and lift your right elbow up toward the ceiling.
- Drop your head back toward the sole of your foot.

WHERE TO ENGAGE:

- Ground down through your pelvis and hips.
- Lift up through your chest.
- Squeeze your elbows and triceps in.

ANATOMY NOTES/ TIPS & TRICKS:

- This is a deep hip opener and backbend. Get comfortable with pigeon and mermaid before attempting this variation.

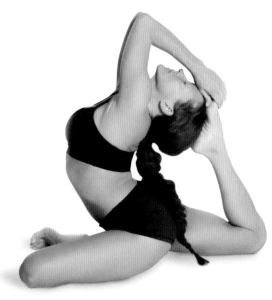

GATEWAY POSE:

LOTUS *(Padmasana)*

Lotus is an intermediate posture that requires flexibility in the hips, ankles, and knees. Sitting in lotus improves hip, knee, and ankle mobility and also assists with posture. For some, lotus may come naturally, but for the majority of people, it's a pose that has to be worked at to master. Try getting comfortable doing one leg at a time before going for the full leg bind.

Lotus is often used as a posture for meditation, and sitting still in the posture can help to improve concentration while also calming and relaxing the mind.

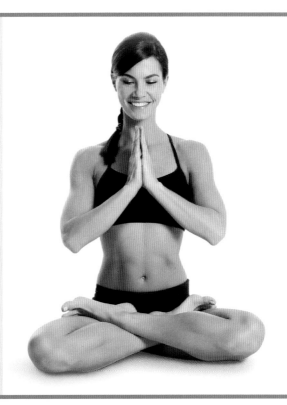

HOW TO GET THERE:

- Start in a seated position.
- Bend your right knee, and bring your right foot toward the top of your left thigh. Work the blade of your right foot into your left hip crease. Use your hand to help you position your foot if needed.
- Bend your left knee, and draw your left foot onto your upper right thigh and upward until it is securely in the lotus position.
- Turn the soles of your feet up to lengthen your ankles.
- Bring your hands to heart center, or rest them on your knees.

WHERE TO ENGAGE:

- Press your ankles down into your thighs.
- Ground down through your pelvis, and lift up through the crown of your head to lengthen your spine.

ANATOMY NOTES/ TIPS & TRICKS:

- This is an advanced hip opening pose that also requires flexibility in your ankles.
- Get comfortable with one leg in the lotus position before attempting the full expression of the pose.
- You will feel a lot of stretch through your feet and ankles.

LOTUS ARM BALANCE:
SCALE *(Tolasana)*

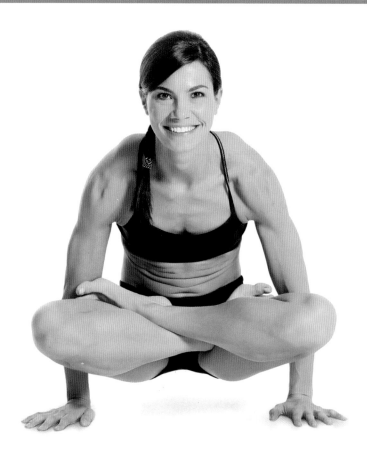

HOW TO GET THERE:

- Begin in lotus.
- Place both palms flat on the floor next to your hips and under your shoulders.
- Press into your palms, straighten your arms, and lift your hips off the floor.

WHERE TO ENGAGE:

- Press your ankles down into your thighs.
- Press firmly into all four corners of your palms and your fingertips.
- Draw your abdominals in and up.

ANATOMY NOTES/ TIPS & TRICKS:

- An engaged and active core is the biggest part of success in holding this pose.
- Be sure your palms are directly under your shoulders to support the weight of your body in the arm balance.

LOTUS ARM BALANCE:
ROOSTER *(Kukkutasana)*

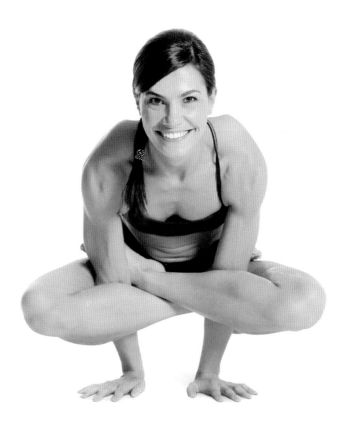

HOW TO GET THERE:

- Begin in lotus.
- Thread your right arm through the space in your right leg between your calf and your thigh. Repeat on your left side.
- Work your legs up as high on your arms as possible.
- Lean forward, press into your palms, and straighten your arms to come into the arm balance.

WHERE TO ENGAGE:

- Press your ankles down into your thighs.
- Press firmly into all four corners of your palms and your fingertips.
- Draw your abdominals in and up.

ANATOMY NOTES/ TIPS & TRICKS:

- The hardest part of this pose is getting your arms through your legs. Use a spray bottle with water or lotion if necessary.
- Trust yourself to lean forward, and bring some weight onto your fingertips.

LOTUS ARM BALANCE:
UPWARD COCK POSE *(Urdhva Kukkutasana)*

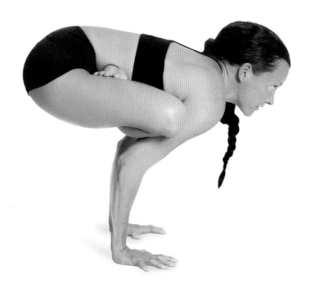

HOW TO GET THERE:

- Begin in lotus.

- Shift weight forward, and come to rest on your hands and knees.

- Place your palms on the floor in front of you in line with your shoulders.

- Bend your elbows slightly, and shift weight forward. Begin to walk your knees up your arms until they rest above your elbows.

- Straighten your arms.

WHERE TO ENGAGE:

- Press your ankles down into your thighs.

- Press into your fingertips.

- Keep your core engaged and drawing in and up.

ANATOMY NOTES/ TIPS & TRICKS:

- This is a difficult pose. An active, lifted core is key.

- Keep flexing through your feet to maintain the lotus position.

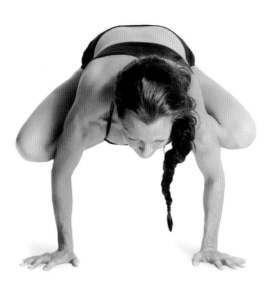

LOTUS ARM BALANCE:
SHORT-TAILED PEACOCK *(Mayurasana)*

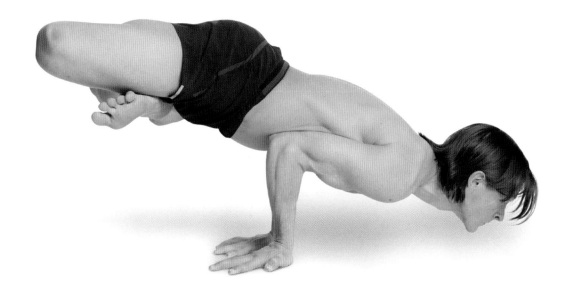

HOW TO GET THERE:

- Begin in lotus.
- Shift weight forward, and come to rest on your knees.
- Place your palms on the mat about 6 inches (15 cm) apart, and turn your fingertips back to face your knees.
- Begin to bend your elbows to 90 degrees, and squeeze your arms into your ribcage.
- Bring your weight and chest forward, and float your legs off the ground.

WHERE TO ENGAGE:

- Press your ankles down into your thighs.
- Press into your fingertips.
- Keep your core engaged.
- Squeeze your upper arms into your ribcage.

ANATOMY NOTES/ TIPS & TRICKS:

- Peacock pose is a difficult arm balance. Be patient finding the right balance of weight between lifting your legs and leaning your upper body forward.
- Your chest will be lower than your legs when starting out, but as you are able, begin to lift your head and chest up to a horizontal position.

Index

ABOUT THE AUTHOR

Jennifer DeCurtins left a six-year career in marketing and advertising in 2011 to pursue yoga, fitness, and writing full-time. She is a registered yoga teacher, NASM certified personal trainer, certified group exercise instructor, CrossFit coach, blogger, and published author. Jennifer is the creator of the popular healthy lifestyle blog *Peanut Butter Runner* where she shares daily updates about food, fitness, and yoga. She's the author of the core training book *Ultimate Plank Fitness: 101 Plank Exercises for a Strong Core, Killer Abs...and a Killer Body.*

Jennifer's yoga practice of choice is vinyasa flow and Ashtanga, and she especially enjoys incorporating back bends, arm balances, and inversions into her practice and classes. She teaches hot power yoga classes in Charlotte, North Carolina, where she lives with her fiance and two golden retrievers.

ACKNOWLEDGMENTS

So much gratitude to my incredible editor Jill Alexander. I admire your vision, creativity, and perseverance. I will never be able to thank you enough for your guidance and dedication in seeing this project come to life. I love teaching yoga more than anything in the world and it's a treasure to have authored this book for yoga students and teachers everywhere.

David Martinell, thank you for taking an overwhelming amount of information and making it so visually dynamic. The book is gorgeous!

Renae Haines, I appreciate your patience and follow through with all the behind the scenes details. Thank you for keeping me on track . . . I know it wasn't always an easy task!

To my photographer, Wanda Koch, only you can make the process of taking hundreds of technical photos full of fun and laughter. It was a joy to partner with you on this project. You are a pillar of our local yoga community and deserve national recognition for your amazing work.

Mom, Dad, and Mema, thank you for supporting my decision to leave the corporate world to follow my passion for fitness, yoga, and writing. Your support and belief means more to me than you'll ever know.

Johnna, participating in your teacher training is what planted the seed for all of these amazing things to happen. I am forever grateful to you for opening the door to self-growth and exploration. It was an honor to showcase your inspiring practice in this book.

Tanner, you see possibility, potential, and light in me that I sometimes cannot see in myself. You constantly push me to keep taking steps that are both scary and exciting, and for that I am grateful. Thank you for the endless hours you spent helping me work on this manuscript and for your assistance with the photography. I would have been lost without you and I think it's safe to say that you somewhat co-authored the book. I am excited about all of the things the future holds for us.

To my students here in Charlotte, in the thousands of hours I have spent in the studio teaching classes, you have taught me just as much as I have taught you. Thank you for your eager, willing spirits, for your vulnerability, and for showing up all in. It is an absolute honor to lead you through practice.